AF412511

CORONARY HEART DISEASE
AND PATTERNS OF LIVING

CORONARY HEART DISEASE AND PATTERNS OF LIVING

ANGELA FINLAYSON and JAMES McEWEN

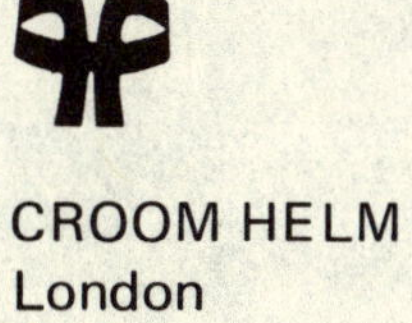

CROOM HELM
London

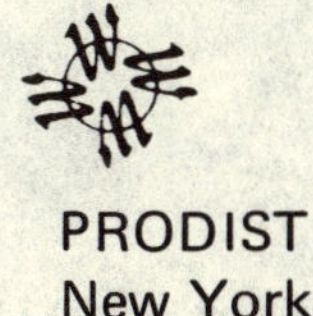

PRODIST
New York

Croom Helm Ltd, 2-10 St John's Road, London SW11

ISBN 0-85664-457-9

First published in the United States by
PRODIST
a division of
Neale Watson Academic Publications, Inc.
156 Fifth Avenue, New York 10010

Library of Congress Cataloging in Publication Data

Finlayson, Angela
    Coronary heart disease and patterns of living.

    Includes bibliographical References
    1. Coronary heart disease – Psychological aspects.
2. Coronary heart disease – Social aspects.
I. McEwen, James, joint author. II. Title.
[DNLM: 1. Life style.   2. Coronary disease.
WG300 F512c]
RC685.C6F48   362.1'96'123   76-56850
ISBN 0-88202-110-9

Printed in Great Britain by Biddles Ltd, Guildford, Surrey

CONTENTS

TO
D.M.F., C.F.F., M.E.F.
A.F.

TO
E.M.M^cE., D.M.M^cE., R.E.M^cE.
J.M^cE.

PREFACE

The study from which information has been drawn to illustrate the theoretical approach adopted in this book was carried out when both authors were working in the Medical Sociology Unit of the Department of Community and Occupational Medicine, University of Dundee.

We wish to express our appreciation to Professor A. Mair and other members of that Department for help and encouragement received in the course of the study. In particular, we would like to acknowledge the detailed advice and practical help with data processing and analysis given by Dr J. Pearson and Mrs C. Murray. Constructive advice at the planning stage was given by Professor R. Illsley, Director of the Medical Research Council Institute of Medical Sociology, Aberdeen. Helpful comments on an earlier version of the text were made by Peter Sheldrake, now Director of the Educational Research and Resources Unit, Flinders University of South Australia. For deficiencies we alone are responsible.

The willing co-operation of hospital consultants, other hospital staff and general practitioners in the Tayside area is gratefully acknowledged.

The material on which this book is based was provided by the patients and their wives who readily invited us into their homes, answered our questions, added explanations and showed deep interest in the enquiry as a whole. In extending to them our sincere thanks, we add the hope that publication in this form will in some way ensure that — as so many of them wished — their experiences will be of value to others.

Support from the Social Science Research Council was received in 1970-72 (by A.F.) in respect of part of the study. Support for secretarial assistance in 1973 was forthcoming from the Chest and Heart Association, Scotland.

The substance of Chapter 12 first appeared in *Social Science and Medicine* (1976), 10, and we thank the editors for permission to use it here.

Numbers varied for different parts of the study and for successive interviews. To avoid excessive detail in the text rounded fractions and percentages are used for the most part, relevant tables being noted in the appendix. More detailed analysis of many of the results is being prepared for submission to specialised journals.

Since total numbers are small, our main conclusions must necessarily be tentative. We hope, however, that in exploring some important aspects of living after myocardial infarction, we have indicated several directions in which other workers in this field — whether in practice or research, and preferably in intervention studies — might move.

1 RECOVERY FROM CORONARY HEART DISEASE IN THE CONTEXT OF CURRENT SOCIOLOGICAL THOUGHT

Our purpose in undertaking this survey was to study the ways in which people cope with the crisis presented by serious illness and with the changes required in the recovery process. Experience of research and teaching in community medicine and in sociology had made us aware of many gaps both in research findings and in the provision of teaching material. Listening to patients and their families had taught us that members of professional services are not always sufficiently conscious of the difficulties encountered in the aftermath of illness nor of the need for deeper understanding and more sustained support. It has therefore been our aim, not only to bridge some of the gaps in research, but to record the process in a way which can be seen as relevant by students and workers in health and social services and also by those concerned with the making of social policy. Since many patients and family members whom we interviewed expressed interest in the survey we hope that they also may feel that we have put their experiences to constructive use.

Within the general area of disability and rehabilitation we were drawn towards the study of recovery from coronary heart disease for several reasons. High incidence, recognition of the fact that it is now increasingly affecting younger persons and lower socio-economic groups, together with the development of new medical techniques which make survival more likely, all combine to present society with a challenge in the provision which it makes for survivors. At the same time, the sudden character of onset affords an opportunity of learning from the experiences of hitherto 'ordinary' individuals and families at a time of stress — 'ordinary' in the sense that they would appear no more likely than anyone else to have pre-existing medical or social problems, and that, unlike patients suffering mental or chronic illness, they and their families would not be expected to have been making gradual long-term adjustments to disability.

Furthermore, the existence of considerable uncertainty permeating the recovery process increases the chances of dissonance in expectations and interpretations arising between patients, families and professionals. On the one hand, current medical emphasis is on 'return to normality' so that the illness has a somewhat marginal status on the spectrum of disability, being often hardly considered as 'disabling' in its consequences; on the other hand, it is frequently felt by patients and families to involve major, long-term adjustments which disturb existing assumptions and patterns of living. These considerations which drew us to the study of recovery from coronary heart disease pointed at the same time to the limitations of the medical model and suggested the need for developing a sociological perspective on the process.[1]

Our approach has been one which encouraged patients and their wives to define the effect of the illness as they saw it and to bring out the problems which seemed most meaningful to them in the recovery period. In adopting this approach we sought theoretical justification from the writings of Thomas,[2] who introduced the concept 'definition of the situation' to emphasise that the individual reacts not just to 'facts' but to his perception of facts and the way in which he perceives will depend on, among other things, his social experience, his expectations for the future, the setting in which he lives, as well as upon the perceptions and meanings which 'significant others' attach to the facts and which they communicate to him.

This concept has been developed by many later writers and the sense in which it has been used by Schutz[3] to include 'recipes for action' seems particularly appropriate for looking at medical regimens from the perspective of patients and families. The crisis may make previous 'recipes for action' no longer tenable, while the recovery process may demand adherence to new 'recipes for action' prescribed by medical services as well as those recommended by rehabilitation services and by 'significant others', who may include employers, spouses and members of social networks. This, in turn, involves redefinition and the making of choices, as Schutz[4] sees it, between different 'projects of action'.

A framework within which this process of redefinition and making of choices can be studied is provided by the concept of 'career' which in recent years has been extended from its occupational source to other areas of behaviour, notably that of mental patients by Goffman,[5] tuberculosis patients by Roth[6] and parents of polio patients by Davis.[7] In such studies the career concept has emphasised the contrast with clinical definitions which tend to concentrate upon one point in time where rehabilitation processes are said to have been successfully or unsuccessfully applied. It can also be used to relate the process of redefinition to different stages of rehabilitation or to different pathways through services and to indicate how taking one pathway rather than another at early turning points may limit subsequent choices.

Applying this concept to recovery from coronary heart disease, we were particularly drawn towards the use recommended by Lemert,[8] not so much to denote fixed stages through which definitions made by patients and their relatives must pass, but to refer to 'recurrent or typical contingencies and problems awaiting patients according to the particular type of career pattern, with the added notion that there may be theoretically "best" choices set into a situation by prevailing technology and social structure'.

This interpretation seemed to accord with our experience in largely unstructured pilot interviews with patients and their wives. They appeared to see the recovery period mainly in terms of difficulties or problems which they had either overcome or, in varying degrees, had failed to overcome. Their attempts to cope with such contingencies could be subsumed as a career, or process, of gradually working out how far new 'recipes for action' could be fitted into existing frames of reference and how far new assumptions and new frames of reference should, and could, be made.

We also came to see the recovery process, or post-infarction career, as necessitating a series of psycho-social transitions comparable in many respects with those described by Fitzgerald in relation to adjustment to blindness[9] and by Parkes in relation to bereavement and other forms of loss.[10] Individuals passing through these transitions have to accept the loss of some roles and some of the ways in which they have hitherto perceived themselves and are required instead to learn new roles and new self-concepts.

Role rearrangement after coronary heart disease seemed likely to be highly problematic in several different ways. While recognising the centrality of the work role to self-identity and social identity for western males in this age group, we sought to balance the dominance accorded to return-to-work in the medical model by focusing also on leisure, family and network roles and on the way in which changes in these roles were seen by wives. Suspecting from pilot interviews that the transition to the role of non-smoker would be very difficult for some patients, we were interested in the implications which this might have for health education, the more so since, unlike most forms of behaviour, smoking is amenable to measurement; the possibility of comparing the smoking habits of

wives with those of husbands both before and after the crisis also
seemed to offer a useful opportunity for studying interaction in a
measurable area.

Changes in an individual's roles and perceptions have to mesh
with changes in the roles and perceptions of 'significant others'.
Hansen and Hill,[11] reviewing the literature on families under various
kinds of stress, have pointed out that what an individual does as
a family member 'largely depends on the expectations that other
members place upon him; the family succeeds only so long as its
members agree on these expectations and try to meet them. Stress
causes change in these role patterns; expectations shift and the family
is forced to work out new patterns.' Croog, Levine and Lurie,[12]
who extensively reviewed the literature on sociological and medical
approaches to the recovery of heart patients, found very few studies
relating recovery level or adjustment of a patient to family-oriented
variables.

We thought it important to discover from wives, not only their
expectations of difficulties but also the resources which they
perceived as available in their social networks for support, in
particular those persons who gave immediate practical help and
those whom they anticipated using as lay consultants. Bott had
suggested using the identification of a woman's helpers at a crisis
as a means of classifying families[13] but, to the best of our
knowledge, this has not been followed up. In this series identification
could be noted not only at crisis but again a year later. We also
wanted to adapt to the post-infarction career some modifications
of techniques used by McKinlay[14] in his study of persons chosen
as lay consultants. This series offered the chance of studying the
extent to which persons chosen as helpers and consultants might
overlap, how patterns might change over a period and, since they
were generally at a later stage in the family life cycle than those
studied by Bott and McKinlay, the effect of the presence in the
network of adult children.

Experience with pilot families had also suggested that we should
supplement the usual objective criterion for outcome in terms of
return/non-return to work by introducing an additional subjective
criterion to distinguish two categories among those returning: that
is, the definition by the wife one year later as to whether or not
the illness was over. This then provided three categories of
outcome: (a) working and illness defined as over; (b) working but
illness defined as not over; and (c) not working.

Finally, we wanted to know whether data collected at first interview with wives, particularly that relating to expectation of difficulties and network resources, would prove to be correlated with outcome and might thus be of predictive value.

Anxieties expressed by wives at first interview proved in general to be well justified. Many men and their wives appeared to have had little scope for making 'best choices'. Right from the beginning many wives seemed to perceive husbands as trapped by unalterable difficulties either in work or personality or both. Often this involved a 'double bind' type of situation whereby, on the one hand, men were expected to 'get back to normal' while at the same time being told that various features in their normal lives were harmful.

Against this general background a relatively small minority emerged at an early stage as having more 'room to manoeuvre' than the remainder. Differences between social classes, age groups and types of family were not clearcut, sometimes reinforcing, sometimes counterbalancing each other. In general they confirmed impressions from pilot interviews that manual workers had most difficulties and poorest outcomes and so did families where the marital roles were 'traditional' rather than 'partnership' in style. To some extent these characteristics went together but not invariably and we were particularly interested in families where atypical patterns prevailed. Youngest workers also appeared to experience many difficulties and poor outcome and this was something which had not emerged in pilot interviews where numbers were small.

We were struck by the minimal use made of services once the men left hospital. This applied overall so could not in itself be said to be an explanation for differences in outcome. However, this lack of contact with professional services meant that the strength of support from informal resources — the family and other members of the social network — was all the more important. Here, congruence — or more often lack of congruence — with professional definitions counted.

While much of the evidence could only be expressed in qualitative terms it did prove possible to quantify some aspects of the post-infarction career. There was evidence of an association between outcome (both objectively and subjectively defined as indicated above) at one year and the range of informal support available. There also appeared to be an association between outcome and the number of areas or domains assessed at first interview as containing potential stressors likely to be still operative in the post-infarction career.

We do not suggest that either of these are causal factors. Rather,

it seems possible that what we were seeing was an illustration of the
'Matthew principle', a cumulative polarisation of fewer difficulties
and greater resources for coping at one extreme and more difficulties
with fewer resources at the other, the two extremes being defined
in terms of a combination of class and outcome. One implication
might be that current emphasis in some of the literature on the 'warm
and supportive' character of close-knit networks could mislead
doctors, social workers and others into too readily assuming that
all such networks can automatically be relied upon to offer sustained
and acceptable support in and after crisis, particularly if the aftermath
requires change in roles and role expectations. Some of the techniques
explored in this study may be applicable to situations resulting from
other illnesses and other forms of crisis, perhaps particularly in
signposting where professional intervention may be most urgently
needed.

Population and Methods

The population was obtained from a consecutive series of men
aged under 60 admitted to four hospital units over a period of
15 months in the early 1970s, who were diagnosed as having sustained
a first myocardial infarction. This diagnosis can sometimes be subject
to doubt but if patients were being treated by the medical staff in
the wards as suffering from myocardial infarction we accepted them
into the series. The study covered all four male medical units in the
city and, since virtually no patients aged under 60 with a diagnosis
of suspected myocardial infarction are treated at home or in a
nursing home, we think that the series is comprehensive. Men who
were single, widowed, divorced or separated were excluded
except in the case of two separated men living in steady cohabitation
who were included; three men refused co-operation for part
or all of the survey; twelve men who were seen in hospital and
whose wives were interviewed at that time died in the following
year.

These exclusions produced a total of 76 men for the main study.
They were seen briefly when in hospital to explain the study and
invite co-operation and interviews were carried out (by JM) at six
months and four years. Wives were interviewed (by AF) at home
(occasionally at place of work or elsewhere) while husbands were
in hospital and again twelve months later. Many of the questions
were pre-coded but interviews were semi-structured to encourage
individuals to expand on areas that were particularly meaningful to

them.

For comparative purposes a simple index of severity was produced comprising state on admission, nature and size of infarction and the presence of complications. On this basis, 22 per cent of patients were considered to be in the 'mild', 48 per cent in the 'moderate', and 30 per cent in the 'severe' category. There was some indication that the younger and older patients were slightly more severely ill, both on admission and on the cumulative index than were those of intermediate ages.

Although the study was concerned with recovery and not with enquiry into causation, except in so far as this was seen by patients and their wives to be relevant, the problems which it raises can only be understood in the context of current medical thought on causation and treatment. This is discussed in Chapter 2, while Chapter 3 brings together medical and sociological perspectives on the concept of rehabilitation and the development of rehabilitation services.

Chapters 4-6 describe the background to the crisis at the time of hospital admission. The following two chapters are concerned with difficulties and changes particularly in relation to medical regimens and work roles as seen by patients at six months. Chapter 9 brings together material on adaptation to role change as seen by patients at six months and by wives at twelve months; smoking habits before and after infarction are reviewed here.

Chapters 10-12 consider wives' perception of problems and coping resources during the year and their definitions of outcome. For administrative reasons it was not possible to carry the study of wives beyond twelve months, a period already longer than that usually covered in follow-up studies. Long-term outcome and definitions made by men at four years are described in Chapter 13. Phases and recurring themes in the post-infarction career are reviewed in Chapter 14 while in the final chapter we discuss possible implications for professional services and for policy. For the most part percentages have been rounded in the text, tables being given in the Appendix.

Notes

1. We were also prompted to this study by already having some experience of the aftermath of coronary heart disease as the by-product of a retrospective study of the association between exposure to asbestos dust and the disease of mesothelioma, in which records of men who had died of heart disease were used as controls and occupational histories were obtained from relatives. (McEwen, J., Finlayson, A., Mair, A. and Gibson, A.A.M. (1970) Mesothelioma

in Scotland. *British Medical Journal* 4, 575-8; Finlayson, A., McEwen, J. and Mair, A. (1971) Home Interviews with Relatives of Deceased Persons. *Scottish Medical Journal* 16, 509-12.) Some of the ideas which we have developed here originated in the course of that enquiry.

2. Thomas, W.S. and Thomas, D.S. (1928). *The Child in America*, New York, Knopf.

3. Schutz, A. (1962). *Collected Papers The Problems of Social Reality* (ed.) M. Natanson, The Hague, Martinus Nijhoff.

4. Schutz, A. (1964). The Stranger. In *Collected Papers II Studies in Social Theory* (ed.) A. Brodersen, The Hague, Martinus Nijhoff.

5. Goffman, E. (1968). *Asylums,* Harmondsworth, Penguin.

6. Roth, J. (1963). *Timetables,* Indianapolis, Bobbs-Merill.

7. Davis, F. (1963). *Passage Through Crisis,* Indianapolis, Bobbs-Merrill.

8. Lemert, E.M. (1967). *Human Deviance, Social Problems and Social Control,* New Jersey, Prentice Hall, p.50.

9. Fitzgerald, R.G. (1970). Reactions to Blindness. An exploratory Study of Adults with Recent Loss of Sight. *Archives of General Psychiatry* 22, 370-79.

10. Parkes, C.M. (1972). What Becomes of Redundant World Models? A Contribution to the Study of Adaption to Change. Paper presented at Third International Conference on Social Science & Medicine, Elsinore (mimeographed).

11. Hansen, D.A. and Hill, R. (1964). Families under Stress. In: Christensen, H.T. (ed.) *Handbook of Marriage and the Family,* Chicago, Rand McNally, p. 806.

12. Croog, S.H., Levine, S. and Lurie, Z. (1968). The Heart Patient and the Recovery Process. A Review of the Directions of Research on Social and Psychological Factors. *Social Science and Medicine* 2, pp. 111-64.

13. Bott, E. (1971). *Family & Social Network: Roles, Norms and External Relationships in Ordinary Urban Families, Reconsiderations,* 2nd ed., London, Tavistock.

14. McKinlay, J. (1973). Social Networks & Utilization Behavior. *Social Forces* 51, 275-94.

2 CORONARY HEART DISEASE : CHANGE AND CHALLENGE IN THE MEDICAL CONTEXT

> Ischaemic heart disease or coronary heart disease has reached enormous proportions, striking more and more at younger subjects. It will result in coming years in the greatest epidemic mankind has faced unless we are able to reverse the trend by concentrated research into the cause and prevention.

Thus the importance of this particular form of heart disease was clearly stated by the World Health Organisation in 1961.[1] The use of the word 'epidemic' emphasises the fact that this is a widespread major disease afflicting the population in general. Epidemic disease never has a single cause. Even with the traditional infectious diseases, the single necessary cause of the infecting organism was never sufficient for an epidemic to occur — cultural, social and environmental factors were always related to the spread of the disease. Epidemics can only occur in a population if there is a confluence of all the causes essential for the widespread development of the disease. It is evident that this is now taking place with coronary heart disease.

The Disease Process

Despite the considerable time, effort and money spent on research into coronary heart disease, many questions still remain unanswered. There appear to be two basic pathological processes involved: (a) atherosclerotic changes in the walls of the arteries supplying the heart muscle; and (b) occlusion of the resulting narrowed lumen of the artery by a thrombus (clot). The deposition of atheroma in the various arteries of the body commencing in early adult life is the fundamental degenerative disorder, but it is only when the supply of oxygenated blood through the coronary arteries is insufficient to meet the demands of the heart muscle, that symptomatic coronary heart disease results. Occlusion of the coronary arteries is not an inevitable result of the process and there is not a precise correlation between the degree of atherosclerosis and clinical coronary heart disease.

The clinical picture is best described as a continuum; it ranges from a symptom-free adult with objective signs of, and evidence of, arterial changes, through one experiencing pain on exercise, to a sudden and unexpected myocardial infarction (heart attack). The classical picture of myocardial infarction due to sudden occlusion of a coronary artery resulting in death of the heart muscle supplied by that artery is easily recognised. Pain similar in nature to anginal pain but of greater severity and unrelieved by rest is accompanied usually by faintness and sweating, and sometimes by vomiting, shortness of breath and a fear of impending catastrophe. There are, however, many possible variants. Occlusion of a main coronary artery may occur without any symptoms at all, particularly in an older person who may have developed a collateral circulation from the other branches of the coronary arteries, sufficient to prevent actual death of a portion of heart muscle. In contrast, myocardial infarction may occur without total occlusion of an artery and for this reason the term myocardial infarction is preferable to the more popular term coronary thrombosis. For simplicity, throughout this book, the term myocardial infarction will be used to describe the sudden event and coronary heart disease will be used for the underlying disease process. This latter term is synonymous with ischaemic heart disease. Thus, those who present with overt evidence of disease point to a much larger group who are asymptomatic, or who either have not recognised or not acted upon symptoms, but in whom the process of atherosclerosis is progressing.

Any attempt to unravel the history of coronary heart disease and the possible factors involved in the causation of the disease illustrates the complexity and the uncertainty that exists. In 1910 in the Lumleian Lectures, Sir William Osler[2] asked questions which are still being asked today: 'Has angina pectoris increased in the community? Has the high pressure of modern days made the disease more common?'

Leibowitz[3] has described in detail the evidence of coronary heart disease in literature. Heberden's description[4] of angina, originally noted by him towards the end of the eighteenth century, could hardly be improved upon today.

> They who are affected with it are seized while they are walking (more especially if it be uphill, and soon after eating) with a painful and most disagreeable sensation in the breast, which seems as if it would extinguish life, if it were to increase or to continue; but the moment they stand still all this uneasiness vanishes.

It is, however, in the present century that the understanding of the condition has advanced and changed most rapidly. This can be illustrated by the writings of Sir James Mackenzie in the early part of this century. In 1913, in *Diseases of the Heart,* Mackenzie[5] believed that angina pectoris was due to exhaustion of the heart muscle but when he wrote *Angina Pectoris*[6] ten years later, he had been convinced by post-mortem studies of patients that the condition was related to coronary disease.

While much dispute has taken place over changes in terminology, changes in medical definition, demographic changes, changes in post-mortem rates and techniques, there is now general belief that coronary heart disease has increased dramatically throughout this century to become one of the most significant causes of mortality and morbidity throughout the world. Some workers consider the increases to be due mainly to an increased incidence of myocardial infarction rather than an increase in the underlying atherosclerotic process, while others, such as Robb-Smith[7], find the evidence for a modern epidemic inconclusive and emphasise the need for greater effort to be made to ascertain the factors involved in the variable individual and ethnic susceptibilities to this condition.

Factors Associated with the Onset of Disease

Sir William Osler's second question on the relationship of the disease to behavioural and environmental factors has proven an even more controversial issue. While it is impossible here to discuss these issues in detail, brief mention must be made of the current understanding of the factors involved in the aetiology of coronary heart disease because many of these factors are intimately related to the individual way of life and may continue to operate in the recovery period. They are also important since attempts may be made to produce alteration in some of them as part of treatment, either to aid recovery or to reduce the risk of further episodes of illness.

Recent studies indicate that people with certain characteristics form a high risk group, in which the chances of death from myocardial infarction are several times greater than in the general population. Coronary heart disease chiefly affects men from the age of forty and its incidence rises sharply with each decade. The condition is less common in women until after the menopause. When the specific factors are discussed later in this chapter it will be seen that many are at least potentially amenable to change, since they are personal or environmental and only a few appear to have a genetic basis.

An illustration of the changing pattern of the disease is shown by comparison of death rates for the different social class categories as defined by the Registrar General. In 1910, from his personal experience, Osler was able to say 'that angina pectoris is an affection of the better classes and not often seen except in private practice'. This belief was supported by the evidence of national statistics until 1951. In the recently published Occupational Mortality Report (1959-1963) for Scotland,[8] it is noted that the standardised mortality ratios by social class for Social Classes I, II, III are almost identical and Social Class IV has the lowest value; this being in contrast to the 1951 Report when there was a downward trend from Social Class I to Social Class V. The recent figures from England and Wales[9] show an even more dramatic change — there now being a positive gradient (i.e. increasing mortality from Social Class I to Social Class V) at ages 15-64. Despite difficulties in comparison, it appears that there is an interesting cohort effect, with the older male cohort having a negative gradient and the younger male cohort a positive gradient. The report suggests that, from this change, a tentative conclusion might be that some factor concerned in the aetiology of atherosclerosis has reversed its social class gradient over the years. Possible factors might be diet, exercise, cigarette smoking or hypertension. The absence of similar changes in the indices for malignant neoplasm of the lung or for hypertension weighs against the last two factors. As Hinkle[10] has suggested, the situation appears to be an increasing incidence of a disease due to 'improved' social conditions.

It is always difficult to determine when an association becomes causal; final proof can only be demonstrated if the disease disappears when the factor under consideration is removed. This is unlikely to be achieved with multifactoral causation, particularly when so many factors are behavioural. Therefore, at present in respect of coronary heart disease we have to be less definite and we are mainly limited to thinking of probable associations. From the results of epidemiological studies in many parts of the world, animal experiments and clinical experience, there is now a vast amount of evidence linking multiple aspects of mode of life with coronary heart disease. These factors are likely to operate over a prolonged period.

At a fairly general level, the most consistent findings are associated with the following risk factors: diet, overweight/obesity; hypertension; tobacco smoking; glucose intolerance (diabetes); sedentary habits; soft water; personality and behaviour; heredity and family history.

In the difficult area of personality characteristics, Caffrey[11] has made important contributions. He considers that, although personality and individual responses to stressful life situations do show some relationship to the development of coronary heart disease, when these individual characteristics are being examined, one should study dimensions of 'normal' behaviour rather than look for psychiatric pathology (extreme neurosis or psychosis) as the distinguishing characteristics of the coronary heart disease victims. He also considers that a distinction should be drawn between those who have angina pectoris alone and those who have myocardial infarction which can be clinically documented. More recently, Gentry and Williams,[12] with a number of other contributors, have produced a valuable summary of the available knowledge of the psychological aspects of coronary heart disease. These contributions warn against too simplistic an approach and perhaps point to the necessity for detailed analysis of factors involved in the different pathological processes. Further work is required to clarify which factors are causal and which are most significant in primary prevention.

Apart from such considerations, attempts have been made to identify and estimate the influence of more specific factors: personal factors such as smoking, diet, physical inactivity, obesity and stress; heredity factors; and environmental factors such as softness of water and occupational conditions. International epidemiological studies point to the likely association between the process of industrialisation in developing countries and a trend towards an increase in coronary heart disease.[12-18]

Whilst the first aim of research must be to elucidate the factors involved in causation and then to seek to introduce programmes designed to prevent coronary heart disease,[19] a widespread primary prevention programme is not an immediate possibility. Indeed, it may be that prevention could only be achieved by radical changes in the life-style of western man. There are signs that, in the realms of diet, physical activity and smoking, positive recommendations are increasingly being made public and there is some evidence of a differential response in the community. In the meantime, considerable effort must be spent in caring for the many people who suffer from coronary heart disease.

The Size of the Problem and its Effects

Britain, and in particular Scotland, has one of the highest rates of coronary heart disease in the world: in Britain, approximately 90,000 men die each year from the disease and in Scotland the figure is approximately 10,000. It is the most important single cause of death representing nearly one quarter of all deaths. Perhaps more informative than these statistics is an understanding of the time scale that may be involved. There has been a tendency to build up the picture of a disease from the basis of hospital statistics, but this provides a very incomplete picture. Community studies[20] such as those in Framingham and Edinburgh have shown that those reaching hospital alive are the survivors of a highly lethal process. Even in a community like Framingham in the United States where a long-term prospective study is being carried out, it appears that fully 40 per cent are not admitted to hospital, as some die too suddenly while, in others, the myocardial infarction is unrecognised. Similar results have been reported from Edinburgh. In summary, for every 100 middle-aged men who have a myocardial infarction, 20 per cent die suddenly, another 20 per cent die in hospital in the first few weeks of the illness and of those who recover, another 20 per cent die within the next five years.

Another way of looking at the size of the problem is to note that approximately fifteen million working days per year are lost on account of the disease. No figures, however, can give a total picture of the cost of a disease in terms of national economy or personal and family suffering.

Although in this study we are concerned with those who survive the initial attack, their quality of life is affected by the general community knowledge of the disease, the current attitude of the medical profession towards acute care and rehabilitation and the widespread uncertainty associated with the condition.

Changes in Care

The pattern of medical care has changed markedly over the past few years from being an essentially negative approach to a positive one. The very fact of this policy reversal presents considerable difficulties and illustrates the problem of innovation and the time lag before there is general acceptance of a change in policy. Many patients and relatives, by virtue of the fact that coronary heart disease is common, have personal experience of the older methods of treatment and know people who have survived (although not necessarily living a 'full' life) after following the older regimen. The new approaches to treatment may appear to them contradictory and hazardous, thus enhancing the uncertainty, fear and conflict already present in the illness situation.

These dilemmas are not limited to the patient and his friends and relatives. Because of the continuing uncertainty regarding causation, it is difficult to offer definitive and rational programmes for prevention and treatment. Thus, tradition, personal prejudices and an attempt to play safe may all influence the doctor's approach.

Price, in 1946,[21] advocated 'at least three months' complete bed rest. . .followed by a similar period of partial rest'. During the ensuing years there has been an increasing tendency towards shorter care but, even ten years ago, there was still an emphasis on absolute

bed rest in hospital for periods ranging from three to six weeks
followed by a very gradual convalescence. Strict instructions, such
as 'take it easy' and 'be careful', were given to the patient, emphasising
what he should not do, with the implication that doing more than was
prescribed might lead to a fatal result. In many cases, this led to a
continuing definition by the patient of being ill and in some dramatic
way, 'different' from his previous 'normal' state. Recovery and
rehabilitation were likely to be limited.

Now the approach is quite different. In many units patients are
sitting in a chair the day following admission, if not severely ill, and
are discharged in under ten days.[22, 23] Nixon[24] describes succinctly
the current positive approach both to the patient with early signs of
coronary heart disease and to those with a sudden myocardial
infarction. He emphasises the importance of active intervention by the
doctor in the early stages in providing information and behavioural
advice to the patient, yet at the same time avoiding unnecessary fear.
With a myocardial infarction there is only one certainty and that is
the importance of early treatment; there is no condition in which it
is more difficult to foretell the future. Since many of the early deaths
are potentially preventable, it is increasingly considered that the patient
should be in a place where the necessary knowledge and facilities are
available. This has led to the development of coronary care units in
hospitals and mobile intensive care units which can provide care at
the earliest stages, prepare the patient for the journey and transport
him to hospital in safety.

In the hospital, depending on the severity of the infarction and
the presence or absence of complications, a wide range of therapeutic
measures may be required — various drug therapies, electric pacemaking
and sometimes surgical treatment. Both in hospital and later, following
discharge, attention must be paid to the patient as an individual, to
his personal and environmental situation, to the factors associated with
the onset of the illness and to the factors resulting from the illness.
Nixon, emphasising that there must be a continuing relationship, writes

> Finally, and with particular regard to the prevention of future
> emergencies the doctor's most useful gift may be to give each
> patient the feeling that he will be welcome for a talk and an
> examination whenever he is overburdened, and that rest and
> protection will be provided whenever a fresh emergency is
> threatened.

Notes

1. World Health Organisation (1969). *Mankind's Greatest Epidemic : Heart Disease*, Resolution and Press Release. Division of Public Information, Geneva, World Health Organisation.
2. Osler, W. (1910). The Lumleian Lecture on Angina Pectoris, Lecture 1, *Lancet* 1, 697-702
3. Leibowitz, J.O. (1970). *The History of Coronary Heart Disease*, London, Wellcome Institute of the History of Medicine.
4. Heberden, N. (1802). *Commentaries on the History and Cure of Diseases*, London, Payne, p. 364.
5. MacKenzie, Sir J. (1913). *Diseases of the Heart*, 3rd edn., London, Hodder and Stoughton.
6. MacKenzie, Sir J. (1923). *Angina Pectoris*, Oxford, Medical Publications.
7. Robb-Smith, A.H.T. (1967). *The Enigma of Coronary Heart Disease*, London, Lloyd-Luke Medical Books.
8. Registrar General For Scotland (1971). *Occupational Mortality (1959-1963)*, Second Supplement to the 114th Annual Report 1968. Edinburgh, HMSO.
9. Registrar General (1971). *Occupational Mortality Tables*. Decennial Supplement; England and Wales 1961, London, HMSO.
10. Hinkle, L.E. (1967). Some Social and Biological Correlates of Coronary Heart Disease. *Social Science And Medicine* 1, 129-39.
11. Caffrey, B. (1967). A Review of Empirical Findings in Social Stress and Cardiovascular Disease. *Millbank Memorial Fund Quarterly* 45, 119-39.
12. Gentry, W.D. and Williams, R.B. (1975). *Psychological Aspects of Myocardial Infarction and Coronary Care*, Saint Louis, the C.V. Mosby Company.
13. de Hass, J.H., Hemker, H.C. and Snellen, H.A. (eds.) (1970). *Ischemic Heart Disease*, Leiden University Press.
14. World Health Organisation (1969). *International Work in Cardiovascular Diseases. 1959-1969*, Geneva, WHO.
15. Social Stress and Cardiovascular Disease (1967). *Millbank Memorial Fund Quarterly* 45, No. 2, Part 2.
16. Rose, G. (1964). Familial Patterns and Ischaemic Heart Disease. *British Journal of Preventive and Social Medicine* 18, 75-80.
17. Morris, J.N., Heady, J.A., Raffle, P.A.B., Roberts, C.G. and Parks, J.W. (1953). Coronary Heart Disease and Physical Activity of Work. *Lancet* 2, 1053-7 and 1111-20.
18. Morris, J.N., Adam, C., Chave, S.P.W., Siren, C., Epstein, L. and Sheehan, D.J. (1973). Vigorous Exercise in Leisure Time and the Incidence of Coronary Heart Disease. *Lancet* 1, 333-9.
19. Joint Working Party Royal College of Physicians of London (1976). Prevention of Coronary Heart Disease. *Journal of the Royal College of Physicians of London* 10, 213-75.
20. Armstrong, A., Duncan, B., Oliver, M.F., Julian, D.G., Donald, K.W. Fulton, M. Lutz, W. and Morrison, S.L. (1972). Natural History of Acute Coronary Attacks. A Community Study. *British Heart Journal* 34, 67-80.
21. Price, F.W. (1946). *Textbook of Medicine*. 7th edn., London, Oxford University Press.
22. Tucker, H.M., Carson, P.H.M., Bass, N.M., Sharratt, G.P., and Stock, J.P.P. (1973). Results of Early Mobilisation and Discharge after Myocardial Infarction. *British Medical Journal* 1, 10-13.
23. Boyle, J.A. *et. al.* Medical Division, Royal Infirmary Glasgow (1973). Early Mobilisation After Uncomplicated Myocardial Infarction. Prospective Study of

538 Patients. *Lancet* 2, 346-9.
24. Nixon, P.G.F. (1973). Coronary Heart Disease and its Emergencies. *The Practitioner* 211, No. 12, 5-16.

3 REHABILITATION : CHANGING CONCEPTS AND PRACTICE

In the medical context three terms which carry slightly different connotations may variously be applied to that stage of the patient career following acute illness — recovery, rehabilitation and resettlement. Recovery is usually taken to indicate the restoration to full health as a natural process aided by therapeutic measures. Rehabilitation implies active measures in addition to normal treatment and is usually applied to patients where there is more serious illness, often with some residual disability, following the acute period and where there may be the possibility of incomplete restoration to health. Resettlement, generally involving employment services, has most frequently been applied to the occupational role but may also be taken to include return to other roles in the community and is seen as the necessary follow on from recovery and rehabilitation. These, however, are not discrete stages nor do all three necessarily occur. There has been some suggestion that, in the context of myocardial infarction, use of the term recovery is, strictly speaking, inappropriate because part of the heart muscle has been destroyed and, although it can be compensated for, it cannot be replaced, so in that sense recovery can never be considered complete. From the perspective of the patient and the family, however, no other term seemed appropriate and accordingly we used it in interview. The term rehabilitation is often used to cover professional intervention in recovery and resettlement and we use it here in this sense, being concerned, on the one hand, with the aims and structure of the rehabilitation services in relation to myocardial infarction and, on the other hand, with the development of sociological thought on the concept of rehabilitation generally.

Rehabilitation for cardiac patients has been defined by the World Health Organisation[1] as 'the sum of activities required to ensure them the best possible physical, mental and social conditions so that they may, by their own efforts, resume as normal a place as possible in the life of the community'.

The World Health Organisation has also attempted to classify the phases of rehabilitation following cardiovascular diseases as follows: (1) at the patients' bedside, involving extensive psychological handling and a phase of light physical rehabilitation; (2) between getting up

and maximum recovery, involving rapid, progressive physical
rehabilitation under continuous clinical and physiological supervision;
(3) direct resettlement with supervision of the patient in his occupational
and social environment or retraining for a new occupation and, during
this stage, measures to maintain his optimum physical capacity are
also introduced.

Although such definitions stress the complexity and diversity of
rehabilitation and consider the individual in his community setting they
give the impression that rehabilitation is a process and a series of steps
rather than a concept. Reference is made to social and family factors
that may hinder rehabilitation but it is assumed that, provided the
right services are available and provided the patient works hard, a
satisfactory outcome will be achieved. Sociological thought, on the
other hand, emphasises that rehabilitation can only be understood in
the context of illness and disability and the meaning which these have
both for individual patients and for society.

Context of Disability

One of the criticisms that has been levelled at Talcott Parsons'[2] concept
of the 'sick role' is that it does not take into account chronic illness,
disability or rehabilitation. However, if it is accepted that there is a
transition from the 'sick role', to the 'rehabilitation role' or the 'disability
role', then his approach appears to be a useful description of one stage
in the career of the disabled person.

The meaning of illness both for the individual who is ill and for those
close to him is generated in social interaction. It is largely dependent,
as we have already seen, on two factors — pre-existing role relationships
(as well as the changes that the illness may produce in these) and the
previous experience of the individual and his family in coping with
difficulties, together with attitudes that have developed during this
process. Prolonged or serious illness transforms the normally short
and temporary 'sick role' into something much more significant and
upsetting. The marked changes that illness can bring about in an
individual's social circumstances have been described by Gordon.[3]
Illness constitutes a frustration of expectations in the individual's
normal life pattern, cutting him off from normal spheres of activity
and disrupting his social relationships to a greater or lesser degree.
Often restricted by an incapacity to function normally, he may have
to learn to live with considerable discomfort or pain and to face severe
alterations to his plans for the future. Indeed his world may very well
appear to be disintegrating.

Adjustment is not helped by the prevailing attitude held by society towards disability. Kessler[4] has described some of the powerful emotions that exist:

> Imperfection in nature is always more or less abhorrent to the human mind. Man has tended to make a fetish of beauty and the human figure is regarded as acceptable only when it is normal. When it is abnormal or deviant in any way from the ideal, the repulsion is equally strong.

The majority of people recovering from serious illness require help and advice from more than one professional area — from general practitioners, hospital doctors, nurses, therapists of different kinds and the specialised skills of psychologists, educationalists and careers advisers. Although, right from the start of the illness episode, the aims of rehabilitation should pervade routine contact with all patients, it may be particularly difficult to initiate such attitudes in hospitals geared to acute admissions, with their emphasis on specialised equipment and patient dependence.

In addition to formal services, the wider environment, particularly the social environment of family, friends, neighbours, staff, fellow patients or rehabilitees and their attitudes and support is known to influence the process of rehabilitation: Lindesmith and Strauss[5] cite studies showing, on the one hand, that friendly interaction with significant others facilitated reestablishment of normal life, while, on the other hand, difficulty in discussing problems with friends led to increasing depression and fear in breast cancer patients.

If rehabilitation is to be seen as a continuing process, there is no justification for assuming that its termination coincides with the end of active treatment. Palmer[6] has shown that, for many patients, discharge from mental hospital is not a joyous homecoming, but the beginning of an isolation more complete than they had experienced in hospital. Even if they manage to find employment and thus an occupational role, they often have no social and family life and accordingly lack other roles. Safilios-Rothschild[7] looks at rehabilitation from three different perspectives. Firstly, she considers rehabilitation at the personality level where the central concept is that of motivation. Secondly, rehabilitation is described in the context of the social system and reciprocal relationships with the various persons involved in the process. Thirdly, rehabilitation is examined at the cultural level; the current form of rehabilitation being related to dominant cultural values. Elsewhere in her study she amplifies some of the

variables that may influence social attitudes: the degree of a country's
socio-economic development and its rate of unemployment; the
prevailing notions about the origins of poverty and unemployment
and socio-political beliefs concerning the proper role of the government
in alleviating social problems; the effectiveness of public relations
groups representing the interests of a specific disability and the dramatic
sensational image attached to a particular illness.

In a similar vein, Strauss[8] cites some evidence suggesting that only
the victims of problems for which remedies were known or anticipated
have been treated sympathetically by their contemporary society.

Being Different and Becoming Deviant

The new very positive approach towards 'return to normality' after
myocardial infarction has been described in Chapter 2. It is necessary
now to consider the implications of 'being different' from 'normal'
either for a short or prolonged period. Since disability, on the whole
(just like illness) has negative consequences for society, it is the definition
of disability as a social problem that results in concern for it as a health
condition. While recognising that there are disadvantages in considering
illness and disability within the context of deviance, we believe that these
are counterbalanced by the insights afforded by the appropriate use of
sociological theory in this area.

Disability can be seen as a form of continuing deviance and a condition
which may be reached in several ways: there may be residual disability
following illness despite the most intensive treatment or the fullest use of
rehabilitation services; there may be a state when achievement is below what
is theoretically possible either because the individual has failed to utilise
the services available or because sufficient and appropriate services may
not be available; the condition may be more or less static or it may fluctuate.

There appear to be two basic pathways: first, one in which there is a
gradual and continuing behavioural transaction between an individual
and significant others until an outcome is reached; and, second, one
in which in a fairly dramatic manner, an individual, without any
action on his part, is suddenly changed and finds himself in a quite
different position. These are the two extremes, but they are not
mutually exclusive. A distinct pathological process may exist in
the first and a behavioural transaction may play a part in the second;
this is especially so in the middle range between the two extremes. The
process in disability is the same as in illness, but it is not reversed as
happens in recovery, being arrested instead.

The principle of primary and secondary deviance as described by

Lemert[9] is fundamental to an understanding of the process. When a person moves from occasional acts of deviance to a life and identity which is organised around the facts of deviance, then he is considered as separated from the rest of society. The importance of the label attached by society will be seen to be of great significance, both the label that the individual attaches to himself and the label that significant others attach to him (the former to some extent being dependent on the latter). The powerful affect of being labelled has been emphasised by Tannenbaum.[10] 'The person becomes the thing he is described as being. Nor does it seem to matter whether the valuation is made by those who would punish or reform.'

Labelling takes place through social interaction and in the case of disability, the interaction is both with the general public and specifically with members of the medical profession. Mercer[11] describes some of the professional characteristics of labelling from a study of the mentally retarded. The clinical perspective tends to perceive deviance as an attribute of the person (as a meaning inherent in his behaviour) and as individual pathology. Individuals assigned to different categories of deviance are compared with each other or with the normal population and appropriate treatment prescribed. There is an assumption that the 'official' definition is somehow the 'right' one and it is generally not queried. Scheff[12, 13] from his study of mental illness, considers that labelling is the single most important cause of careers of continuing deviance.

Whether the entry to the state of deviance is slow or rapid and whatever the reasons, there then follows a stage of confirmation: the individual comes to learn the mores, the values, the attitudes, the rules, the patterns of behaviour and the jargon of his new subculture. He becomes accepted by the people of that community as a fellow member and once he has been so labelled, self-awareness is forced upon him and he must face the fact that he is a particular type of person, in this case a disabled person. The process of socialisation to this new role is more dramatic if he is publicly or officially labelled through hospitalisation or other medical contact. The individual is intimately involved in this process of conversion and gradually comes to accept that he is what others see him to be; he does not play the new role fully until he has been identified in that role by others or by himself and has thus become committed to it.

Stigma and Stereotypes

Goffman[14, 15] has described stigma as referring to an attribute that

is deeply discrediting. He emphasises, however, that this is a language
of relationships, rather than of attributes, since an attitude that
stigmatises one type of possessor can confirm the usualness or point
to the exceptional value of another and therefore is neither creditable
nor discreditable as a thing in itself. The stigmatised individual becomes
reduced in the mind of the observer from a whole or usual person to
a tainted and discredited one.

Many factors are relevant in the development of an individual's
attitude towards deviance — the generally held cultural attitudes in
the particular society to the specific form of deviance, his moral
evaluation of the cause leading to the deviance and the knowledge
that he has of people with the particular form of deviance.

The importance of society's labelling role has been described
but Goffman elaborates this, pointing to the way in which society,
at one and the same time, tells the stigmatised individual that he is
a member of the wider group which means that he is a normal human
being, but that he is also 'different' in some degree and that it would
be futile to deny the difference.

Closely allied to the way that stigma develops is the way in which
stereotypes of deviance are built up. The stereotypes tend to be of
extreme types; in addition to a general picture of a deviant, specific
subdivisions arise for different kinds of deviance including stereotyped
images of the drug addict, the alcoholic, the schizophrenic, the epileptic,
the blind man and the man who has had a 'heart attack'. There is a
tendency to assume that anyone who falls into one of these categories
has all the attributes of the stereotype. The characteristics of abnormality
are emphasised and the characteristics of normality forgotten.

Self-conceptions in Disability

The attitudes that the individual develops towards his disability
may be related less to its severity than to his previous personality and
social experience and the way in which he interprets its effect on his
total social functioning, including the requirements of his occupation.

Litman[16] describes from his own study and from other published
works, some of the self feelings that may develop in a disabled person:
(1) fear that it is not himself as a person but his injury that is of primary
importance to others; (2) fear that the injury devalues him as a person;
(3) guilt connected with the feeling of being a burden; (4) conflict
between the desire for dependence and independence; (5) feelings of
self pity.

Litman has also drawn attention to some findings which seem to be

at variance with some widely held concepts about disability. These
have important implications for rehabilitation, and perhaps particularly
after myocardial infarction, since it seems that: (1) an overt or visible
injury does not necessarily have more of an effect upon self-concept
than a non-visible injury or illness; (2) amputees can more readily
evaluate their abilities and their disabilities than those with a generalised
illness; (3) a physical loss seems to be incorporated into the self-concept
more adequately and with less general damage than an all-pervasive
illness.

Outcome of Deviance

Even when there has been commitment to the deviant role, it does
not follow that further change is impossible. New roles may be learned
and adopted, the disability may be altered by new treatment; new
interactional situations may develop and former roles may be reassumed.
Lemert[9] points out, however, that the cost in terms of time, energy and
distress to achieve this may be considered by the deviant to be too high.

Another factor of significance in the maintenance of deviant
identity is reward and punishment, which is closely related to the
influence of agencies and organisations. Labelled deviants may be
rewarded for playing the stereotyped deviant role and they may be
punished when they attempt to return to normal, or more conventional,
roles. This is well illustrated in the field of mental illness. Mechanic[17]
has shown the importance which staff attach to getting the patient to
accept the psychiatric definition of his condition, refusal sometimes
being taken as a further indication of his illness. Scheff[12] has described
ways in which patients who show insight into their mental illness are
rewarded by psychiatrists. Similarly Roth[18] has illustrated these points
in his work on rehabilitation including recovery in the hospital situation
and other careers. Rewards may simply consist of staff approval or they
may involve a variety of forms of personal satisfaction for the
individual. Lemert[9] illustrates how an individual may be torn between
the desire to rid himself of the stigma attached to a particular condition
and the secondary rewards associated with the particular form of deviant
behaviour or disability.

A possible legitimised outcome is the 'disabled role': Haber and
Smith[19] in their account of disability as a social process, describe the
interaction between the individual and society which will lead to
a normal adaptation to incapacity; the accredited disabled individual
will develop patterns of acceptable behaviour which have themselves
become normalised, being seen as alternative patterns of behaviour

expected in respect of that particular disability.

It is important to distinguish between the given physical limitation that a particular illness imposes and the individual's total functioning. Individuals react in many different ways to particular limitations and a wide variety of coping mechanisms are called into play, much depending on a particular individual's previous social functioning including the requirements of his occupation and his social and leisure pursuits. Mechanisms range all the way from complete denial of the condition and refusal to recognise its effects, accompanied by a refusal to give in to it or acknowledge the need for help, to, at the other extreme, complete dependence, unrealistic demand for help and a total rejection of all attempts by others to encourage self-help. Sometimes, associated with the latter there may be a full acceptance by the patient of all the secondary gains of illness, including exemption from normal role obligations, acceptance of multiple sources of help and full use of the sick role in bargaining and negotiation.

Role Transition

Szasz and Hollander[20] have described three models of doctor-patient interaction which can serve as a basis for examining the role transition which is necessary in rehabilitation. The models are: Activity-Passivity — the physician 'actually does something to the patient' who acts only as a 'passive recipient'; Guidance-Co-operation — the physician 'tells the patient what to do and the patient acts as co-operator'; Mutual Co-operation — the physician 'helps the patient to help himself' and the patient acts as an active participant in the partnership. It is not suggested that these reflect clear-cut distinctions between stages in rehabilitation. Some aspects of rehabilitation may appear in the very early stages of treatment of illness, e.g. physiotherapy to the passive and dependent patient, and some aspects of treatment may carry through to the late stages of rehabilitation, e.g. drug therapy for angina, hypertension or ectopic beats.

Rehabilitation, however, should not be thought of as something that is applied to a patient like drug therapy or a surgical procedure performed by a doctor on a passive patient but as an active process of participation by the individual (preferably no longer considered a patient) in a series of activities suited to his individual needs. Both the patient and the doctor must assume new roles if the process is to be successful. Both must see the sick role as temporary. At present, there is a tendency for the medical profession to assume that a person is either sick or well, and that the need for rehabilitation implies that he must be sick. Thus an individual may be forced both by professional attitudes and the present structure of medical rehabilitation services to continue in the sick role.

Safilios-Rothschild[2] stresses the importance of 'being an agent of change' rather than a passive object in the hands of the rehabilitation team. Those closely linked to the individual both in the hospital setting and when he returns to the community must recognise and be involved in the process of role transition.

Keith[21] has put forward a plan for a new model for rehabilitation based on this change of role. In the old model, rehabilitation takes place in a medically oriented centre where patients are required to renounce whatever remaining autonomy they possess; goals are usually set with little involvement of patients or families; patients are expected to rise and to go to bed at set hours and to adhere to prescribed schedules; they are also expected to contribute hard work without questioning the treatment routines of physical and occupational therapy and cannot leave the centre without permission from the medical authorities. In contrast to this, Keith puts forward the 'maximum independence model'. Every aspect of the individual's range of competence would be reviewed with him and activity would be related to agreed levels to avoid assignment to a routine likely to encourage dependence. Free communication of information both to him and his relatives and full participation by the latter in any decision that concerns him would be directed at reducing gaps between staff and individuals in their expectations of outcome. There would also be regular reassessment and full discussion of all procedures being used.

Although measures such as these represent a great advance on older thinking there are still many uncertainties about how best to help people through difficult role transitions. Rose[22] believes that there are some barriers to rehabilitation and that success may be limited. He suggests that a person can never 'unlearn' something, although he can drastically modify the learning. A concept of self, once learned, affects an individual's behaviour throughout his life. New self-concepts may be learned but the old is never forgotten and the ensuing behaviour is the outcome of the struggle between the old and the new self-concept:

> If an individual for example, once conceives of himself as an alcoholic, a drug addict, a criminal or whatever, he will never completely eliminate that self-concept, and even if he were to be 'cured' by learning

new self-concepts, a temptation to take a drink, or drug, or steal something will have a challenging meaning for such an individual which it does not have for another individual who has never defined himself as an alcoholic, a drug addict or criminal.

To help himself through the difficult process of role transition, the patient learns to use a strategy of negotiation or bargaining. Just as he largely takes the initiative in deciding when to seek medical help, so he is to some extent responsible for the decision to terminate this relationship. During recovery he is either given or demands back control over the parts of his life which he had ceded to others (nurses, doctors, family) during the acute stages of illness. He gradually resumes his normal social obligations and gives up the special privileges of the sick role. This process is made more complex by the fact that, in the same way as both patients and doctors have built up stereotypes of illness, so they have concepts of what certain disabilities are like, how long they last and what is the normal recovery time. Thus both have yardsticks against which to measure progress. As with virtually all varieties of biological and social norms the range is wide, differences being accentuated by diverse patterns of socialisation so that the professionals (doctors, nurses, therapists) on one hand and the patient and his relatives on the other, may be working from entirely different bases of knowledge and power. Thus the scene is set for negotiation over many aspects of recovery and rehabilitation.

Negotiation over timetables has been described by Roth[18] in his study of tuberculosis hospitals. Many of his findings can be applied to other conditions equally well. Each patient attempts to find out how long his treatment is likely to last by comparing himself and his condition with other patients and, for their courses of treatment, estimates what is a likely period for himself. As a group, the patients develop time norms, against which each individual patient can measure his progress. The staff also have their 'normal timetables' built up from their past experience which, in turn, influence patients. The patients are always concerned to ascertain the minimum timetables for treatment, while, to the staff, timing is less important and they bring other factors, usually of a technical nature, into their decision-making. Roth[18] points to the development of conflict between doctors and patients because they are using different sets of categories, those of the doctor being more highly differentiated than those of the patient. Bargaining occurs because the patient is constantly pressing for advancement of the timetable while the doctor may resist this as his criteria may indicate that the time for less restriction and advancement to the next stage of treatment has not yet been reached. This process, however, does enable the patient to break up what would otherwise seem to be a long and indefinite sentence by means of recognised bench-marks and so to structure the progress of his recovery.

Other aspects of negotiation in recovery have been studied by Davis[23] in families where a child developed poliomyelitis. He drew attention to the attempts by parents to obtain knowledge of their child's condition and of the degree of disability that might be expected. The failures in communication, the frustration and the different relationships which developed with different staff members and with the community illustrated many problems of negotiation that arise in the recovery situation.

Rehabilitation Services in Britain

Until recently rehabilitation has been regarded as a fringe speciality and yet many doctors would consider it as an integral part of daily medical care. Writing in 1970, Yates[24] claimed that the rehabilitation services for the disabled in Britain were potentially the best in the world. All the services were there, yet total achievement fell short of their collective objective owing to lack of co-ordination. He considered that the administrative structure was comprehensive but so complex that the disabled person could find himself shunted from pillar to post because of departmentalism.

Many reports have, in fact, indicated that services which followed after acute medical or surgical care often lacked equivalent quality or efficiency and thus full recovery may be either delayed or not achieved. In Scotland, studies[25,26] published in the 1950s and early 1960s showed quite clearly that there was a failure to obtain maximum benefit from existing services.

At present, relatively few patients attend any formal rehabilitation establishments and rehabilitation is only likely to be considered if the patient has some obvious problem or specifically requests contact with a relevant specialist. Occupational difficulties are usually the presenting problem but referral may be suggested by a ward sister, houseman, consultant or social worker; alternatively, the patient or a relative may ask for an appointment with the medical social worker.

In some hospitals, resettlement clinics exist where representatives of a number of different professions gather with the patient to discuss problems. They usually consist of the specialists together with the general practitioner, the hospital social worker and the disablement resettlement officer of the Employment Service Agency. Here, initial assessment can be undertaken and a path of action initiated Where such clinics do not exist the patient may be referred directly to a medical rehabilitation unit or to the disablement resettlement officer at the local office of the Employment Service Agency. Medical rehabilitation units may either be general or related to a specific type of disability; they may be either residential or designed for daily attendance; similarly some Employment Rehabilitation Centres (ERCs) are residential and severity of disability is usually the determining factor in allocation.

Difficulties in communication between services are increased by the fact that these services are run by different government departments. Some patients may be recommended for retraining by ERCs and then pass to a Government Skill Centre for specialist training suited to their residual disability. Even within the health service difficulties in communication may arise; this is especially likely in respect of those patients who require transfer from one unit to another and is also likely to affect a high proportion of patients at the time of discharge from hospital to the community. Where difficulties are complex other services may also be involved, including those run by local authorities especially social work departments, as well as other organisations, some statutory, others voluntary, which may be required to deal with specialised aspects such as housing, legal and financial arrangements. For individuals with multiple problems, the necessary co-ordination of services may be feasible only within a rehabilitation unit specifically oriented to their needs; for those requiring fewer or simpler services, it is still desirable that some professional person should be charged with assessing just what these needs are likely to be and guiding them to the appropriate services in the community.

Rehabilitation has been very inadequately taught in most British medical schools and little has been done to encourage the doctor to enter the field of rehabilitation. Recently, two committees, one in England, under Professor Sir Ronald Tunbridge,[27] and one in Scotland, under Professor A. Mair,[28] have produced reports which have stimulated interest in this field. The Scottish Committee's Report emphasised, *inter alia,* that: medical rehabilitation should be recognised as a speciality in its own right and academic aspects must be developed both at postgraduate and undergraduate levels; considerable opportunities for research exist in respect of medical assessment, work assessment, the interrelationship of health and social work services and other aspects of rehabilitation services; special attention should be paid to the co-ordination of services, the provision of suitable accommodation, including day hospital facilities, and the development of information services about aids and appliances; and that voluntary organisations, having a continuing essential role to play, must work more closely together and in association with statutory bodies

It is hoped that these recommendations, together with developments in community medicine, and changes in the organisation of health and social services will lead to a considerable improvement in attitudes towards rehabilitation and to more comprehensive and suitable care being established for all the patients who require it.

Rehabilitation after Myocardial Infarction

We can now turn from the general context within which rehabilitation services operate in contemporary Britain to consider factors more specifically related to myocardial infarction and to the conditions prevailing in Dundee at the time of this study. It is against this background that the post-infarction careers of the men in this series should be seen.

As noted in Chapter 2, there has been, over the past decade, a considerable change in emphasis in medical thought with the realisation that, following myocardial infarction, inactivity is usually more harmful than activity and, in particular, that for men of working age, return to work (although possibly changed work) in many cases is both desirable and feasible. As part of this more positive approach, it is now usually expected that, provided there are no serious complications, patients are physically fit enough to be working six months after onset; indeed many doctors now expect this earlier. As with all innovation, however, progress occurs at an uneven pace and changed attitudes do not always match changes in knowledge and policy. Among factors hindering full implementation of the new approach, Levine[29] has diagnosed 'physician fear', that is, the doctor's fear of being blamed if a patient dies. He is seldom blamed for patients who die in their beds, particularly if he has given a pessimistic prognosis, but he may be blamed if they die after he has encouraged them to be active. Levine believes that an optimistic approach by the doctor rarely does harm in comparison with the mental suffering and the loss both of earning power and of quality of life which he considers often result from unnecessary restraints applied to some cardiac patients. In similar vein, Clark[30] suggests that, in most instances, the physician requires above all an enlightened, fearless and optimistic approach and a refusal to procrastinate, particularly with regard to return to work.

Another circumstance which may have operated against full implementation of the changed approach is the absence in Britain of specialised follow-up clinics or rehabilitation services specifically for post-infarction patients. In some European countries, particularly Scandinavia, Holland and Eastern Europe, there are specialised work assessment units where detailed analysis of cardiac patients' abilities and disabilities are made and appropriate schedules of physical training carried out, usually with specific reference to the work situation. These may be accompanied by various forms of individual or group psychotherapy, sometimes including other family members. Similar programmes are frequently found in the USA. At the time when this study was carried out in Dundee the general facilities described were available but no specialised ones existed. Recently published reports[31,32] have been more positive and more specific in their recommendations.

Failure to provide such specialised facilities in Britain may have been encouraged by previous reports suggesting that apparently good results occur without them. Most studies show that 60 to 80 per cent of patients who have survived the acute illness return either to their former employment or to a changed type of work with reasonably good long-term survival. It has also been shown that patients who return to work following the acute episode are no more frequently off work for short spells of 'sickness absence' than others nor is there a higher incidence of industrial accidents. Where it has so far been possible to assess the first results of the new policy of early and active rehabilitation, this has suggested lower mortality and a lower incidence of complications.

Such studies, however, have used only medical models for assessment of results — lowered mortality, return to work, absence of recorded complications. They ignore the possibility that the two latter criteria may conceal much impairment of the quality of life both for the patient himself and for his family.

It has been said of rehabilitation that the task 'is not to add years to life but life to years'. Another perspective is to consider rehabilitation, paradoxically, as a form of prevention. When an illness has not been prevented (by primary prevention) and has not been cured (by secondary prevention), it can still be prevented (tertiary prevention) from becoming an incapacitating condition and, possibly, the chance of recurrence or further development of the condition can be reduced if not eliminated.

It was largely because we were aware of discrepancies between the results as judged by purely medical criteria and the lasting impact

which myocardial infarction can be seen to have on patients and their
families that we embarked on this study which, while utilising accepted
medical criteria, attempts to complement these by also taking into
account subjective criteria which have a validity of their own when
seen in the framework of current sociological thought.

Notes

1. World Health Organisation (1969). *Rehabilitation of Patients with Cardio-Vascular Disease. Report of a Seminar, Hanover, 1967.* Copenhagen, Regional Office for Europe, Euro 0381.
2. Parsons, T. (1951). *The Social System,* New York, The Free Press.
3. Gordon, G. (1966). *Role Theory and Illness: A Sociological Perspective,* New Haven, College and University Press.
4. Kessler, H.H. (1953). *Rehabilitation of the Physically Handicapped,* New York, Columbia University Press.
5. Lindesmith, A.R. and Strauss, A.L. (1968). *Social Psychology,* 3rd edn., New York, Holt Rinehart and Winston.
6. Palmer, M.B. (1958). Social Rehabilitation for Mental Patients. *Mental Hygiene* 42, 24-8.
7. Safilios-Rothschild, C. (1970). *The Sociology and Social Psychology of Disability and Rehabilitation,* New York, Random House.
8. Strauss, R. (1965). Social Change and the Rehabilitation Concept. In: Sussman, M. (ed.) *Sociology and Rehabilitation,* New York, American Sociological Association.
9. Lemert, E.M. (1967). *Human Deviance, Social Problems, and Social Control,* New Jersey, Prentice Hall.
10. Tannenbaum, F. (1968). The Dramatization of Evil. In: Rubington, E. and Weinberg, M.S. (eds.) *Deviance. The Interactionist Perspective,* London, Collier-MacMillan.
11. Mercer, J.R. (1965) Social System Perspective and Clinical Perspective: Frames of Reference for Understanding Career Patterns of Persons Labelled as Mentally Retarded. *Social Problems* 13, 21-30 and 33-4.
12. Scheff, T.J. (1963). The Role of the Mentally Ill and the Dynamics of Mental Disorder : A Research Framework. *Sociometry* 26, 436-53.
13. Scheff, T J. (1966). *Being Mentally Ill; A Sociological Theory,* Chicago, Aldine.
14. Goffman, E. (1968). *Stigma,* Harmondsworth, Penguin.
15. Goffman, E. (1968). *Asylums,* Harmondsworth, Penguin.
16. Litman, T.J. (1962). Self-Conception and Physical Rehabilitation. In: Rose, A.M. (ed.) *Human Behavior and Social Process: An Interactionist Approach,* London, Routledge and Kegan Paul.
17. Mechanic, D. (1962). Some Factors in Identifying and Defining Mental Illness. *Mental Hygiene* 46, 66-74.
18. Roth, J.A. (1963). *Timetables,* Indianapolis, Bobbs-Merrill.
19. Haber, L.D. and Smith, R.I. (1971). Disability as Deviance : Normative Adaptations of Role Behavior. *American Sociological Review* 36, 87-97.
20. Szasz, T. and Hollander, M.H. (1956). *A Contribution to the Philosophy of Medicine. The Basic Models of Doctor-Patient Relationship,* AMA Archives of Internal Medicine 97, 585-92.
21. Keith, R.A. (1968). The Need for a New Model in Rehabilitation. *Journal of Chronic Diseases* 21, 281-6.
22. Rose, A.M. (1962). A Systematic Summary of Symbolic Interaction Theory.

In: Rose, A.M. (ed.). *Human Behavior and Social Process. An Interactionist Approach,* London, Routledge and Kegan Paul.
23. Davis, F. (1963). *Passage Through Crisis,* Indianapolis, Bobbs-Merrill.
24. Yates, G. (1970). *Rehabilitation Services for the Disabled,* London, Report to the Nuffield Foundation.
25. Ferguson, T. and MacPhail, A.N. (1954). *Hospital and Community,* London, The Nuffield Provincial Hospitals Trust. Oxford University Press.
26. MacKenzie, M., Weir, R.D., Richardson, I.M., Mair, A., Harnett, R.W.F., Curran, A.P. and Ferguson, T. (1962). *Further Studies in Hospital and Community,* London, The Nuffield Provinical Hospitals Trust. Oxford University Press.
27. Tunbridge, Sir R. (Chairman) (1972). *Rehabilitation* Report of a Sub-committee of the Standing Medical Advisory Committee, London, HMSO.
28. Mair, A. (Chairman) (1972). *Medical Rehabilitation : The Pattern for the Future,* Report of a Subcommittee of the Standing Medical Advisory Committee, Edinburgh, HMSO.
29. Levine, S.A. (1960). Physician's Fear : A Deterrent to Rehabilitation among Cardiacs. *Geriatrics* 15, 534-42.
30. Clark, R.J. (1960). Rehabilitation of the Cardiac Patient — Employment and Cardiac Impairment. *Geriatrics* 15, 529-33.
31. Royal College of Physicians of London and the British Cardiac Society (1975). Cardiac Rehabilitation 1975. Report of a Joint Working Party. *Journal of the Royal College of Physicians of London* 9, 282-346.
32. International Society of Cardiology, (1973). *Myocardial Infarction. How to Prevent. How to Rehabilitate.* Handbook of the Council, Mannheim, Boehringer.

4 FIRST MYOCARDIAL INFARCTION : START OF — OR STAGE IN — THE PATIENT CAREER?

The discussion in Chapter 2 on the underlying disease process has indicated that, although the onset of a myocardial infarction may be sudden, it is not necessarily a totally unexpected or chance outcome. Never the less, many people — patients, family, friends and doctors — emphasise the sudden and unexpected nature of the event. They might hardly expect, therefore to find any discussion of such processes as normalisation of symptoms, delay in seeking medical help, or the influence of social and psychological characteristics, which usually serve as preludes to sociological approaches to illness. In contrast to the situation in chronic or mental illnesses, first myocardial infarction seems to offer an illustration of a patient career with a clear-cut beginning, at least from the patient's perspective and his experience of being suddenly defined by others as dangerously ill. Indeed, it might be considered as one of the most dramatic onsets to a patient career. Did the experience of this series confirm this? At first sight it seemed to do so. 'Such a shock', 'Out of the blue', 'We never thought', were typical comments made by patients and their wives. It soon became clear however, that the sense of sudden shock meant that the 'heart attack' was unexpected and not necessarily that their previous state of health had been seen as satisfactory.

Evidence is gradually accumulating from a number of studies that many infarctions are preceded by a period during which patients experience a variety of conditions ranging from defined ill-health to vague malaise. This has very important implications for society at large, as well as for patients, their 'significant others' and professionals, forcing us to look again at the two main theoretical concepts used in this study. First, we are required to re-examine the use of patient career in the light of coronary heart disease as a condition with a wide variety of modes of onset as opposed to considering only the dramatic and sudden onset generally associated with a myocardial infarction. Although, for many in this series, the infarction is a dramatic episode in a pre-existing illness career, it is not an identical event in a series of identical careers. Second, it draws attention to the importance of the definitions that are attached to this preceding period of ill-health or malaise by the individuals involved — the patient, 'significant others' and doctors — as well as the action which results from these definitions.

Exploration of this phase is the more difficult because, as many writers have pointed out, feeling unwell is not an unusual state. A recent study by Wadsworth[1] found 95 per cent of South Londoners considering themselves as unwell during the two week period before questioning. Moreover, it is known that, retrospectively, especially after a crisis, people tend to reorder their experience and may select only those features which appear to fit their current understanding of causation. Accepting these difficulties, we still thought that some enquiry should be made into the pre-infarction career as seen by the patient and his wife. This was partly because any interpretations which they made about causation seemed likely to be carried over into their expectations and interpretations concerning post-infarction contingencies, particularly if it was thought that some detrimental factor was likely to continue to be operative; and partly because their attitudes and behaviour in, for instance, the processes of normalisation and help-seeking could suggest how they might respond to post-infarction contingencies. So we looked particularly for evidence of ways in which normal social functioning had been disturbed and how it was brought to the attention of others and how interpreted.

Other studies have distinguished more than one pattern in the preceding phase, of which the most easily recognised is that where patients have already been defined as suffering from angina of effort. In this series, Table 4.1, angina had been diagnosed in only one in every ten, although nearly as many again had symptoms associated with other forms of heart disease such as raised blood pressure. This figure is low in comparison with the findings of Short and Stowers[2] in Aberdeen who found that, in just over one half of those who developed coronary heart disease, the first symptom was angina. Their figures represent the result of a meticulous review of a wider range of patients whereas our one in ten refers only to those who had sought professional advice and to whom the diagnostic label had been specifically applied. Short and Stowers emphasise the difficulty that exists in recognising the symptom, particularly when it is localised in an unusual site, when its occurrence is dependent on a combination of exercise with cold or a recent meal or when it is induced by excitement rather than effort.

Angina may progress to the second condition which has been defined as the Pre-infarction Syndrome, when any of the following factors are present: (1) recent onset of crescendo angina; (2) recurrence of crescendo angina after a symptom-free period; (3) sudden change of angina pattern with reference to increasing frequency, or lack of response to trinitrate; (4) sudden development of angina at rest or during sleep. Several patients in our series presented this picture, but usually only for a very short period prior to the actual infarction with which it is easily confused.

Perhaps the most interesting and controversial category consists of those patients with ill-defined symptoms. In this series, just over one half considered that they had been generally unwell before infarction, approximately one in every five claiming to have experienced symptoms for between one and thirty days; a similar proportion claiming symptoms having lasted between one month and one year; and the remainder asserting that these had been present for more than a year. Nearly one quarter went to the extent of defining themselves as ill in the period preceding the infarction, and, altogether, less than one third claimed to be totally symptom-free immediately before infarction. This accords well with other studies, which show that prodromal symptoms including retrosternal pressure, sensation or pain, arm aches, excessive fatigue and choking sensation, are detected in up to four out of every five patients with well documented myocardial infarction. Many patients interpret these prodromal symptoms as manifestations of indigestion and not infrequently take various kinds of antacid remedies for relief.[3] In some of this series, symptoms amounted to no more than brief attacks of chest tightness and choking; one such episode, eleven months before infarction, was subsequently recognised by the patient as a milder version of what he later learned to define as heart disease.

These diffuse symptoms, especially tiredness, present considerable diagnostic problems as they can be associated with virtually any disease process as well as often being accepted as a normal expectation. From the medical perspective it has been suggested that emphasis should be on the recognition of *abnormal* tiredness and its effects on the functioning of the individual. Nixon[4] describes this as follows:

There is an abnormal tiredness which can overcome the will of the active and aggressive person and either modify his activities or provide him with an increasing struggle to maintain his customary habits. Irritability, accelerated ageing and the jettisoning of spare-time activities are often very worrying to wives but pride causes the patient to conceal the deterioration which is aggravating his insecurity.

Normalisation of Symptoms

Although Nixon[4] has indicated that prodromal symptoms influence a person's normal social functioning it is often difficult to determine the extent of this. Rather than the fairly clear-cut picture which he paints, evidence from this series suggested that the diffuse, intermittent, non-visible character of early symptoms meant that, until they reached a very acute stage, they did not interfere with occupational functioning, so no one in the work setting or outside the nuclear family had any reason to define men as ill. Mechanic[5] has pointed out that, under conditions of manageable difficulties, persons have a tendency to normalise or ignore symptoms that do not become too severe. For these men, difficulties appeared manageable as long as they were able to continue in the occupational roles with which they closely identified themselves. Pain or discomfort could be attributed to indigestion, ulcers, strained muscles, arthritis. Conditions such as tiredness or irritability could be accepted as a normal accompaniment to hard work. (Robinson[6] has pointed out that manual workers, in particular, accept tiredness as a normal expectation or as part of the ageing process.) In such ways, men appeared to have been normalising symptoms over varying periods of time.

Many previous studies, for instance, that of Yarrow[7], dealing with normalisation of symptoms, have been made within the context of mental illness, in which resistance by patients and families to the definition is compounded by reluctance to accept the stigma associated with it. This concentration on mental illness has perhaps caused neglect of the normalisation process in other forms of illness. It may be of relevance that, during pilot studies, we received a detailed written account of her husband's pre-infarction symptoms from a woman who described the eventual diagnosis of coronary thrombosis as coming almost as a relief since, until that moment, she had been fearing, although not admitting to herself, that he was approaching mental breakdown.

Altogether, four out of every five women mentioned some condition such as husbands seeming 'out of sorts', 'off colour' or 'just not right' but these conditions were not of a kind that they could easily identify. Many explained that their husbands considered such conditions to be temporary or trivial or both, as these examples show:

For the past year everything has seemed a difficulty — the sweat would pour down his forehead over little things. Last year was the worst but in the past two years, he has aged a lot. Its natural to be getting older but it was happening too rapidly. I used to suggest he should see a doctor about his varicose veins and he was always going to go but when you've your own business you're inclined to put it off — its years since he saw a doctor.

He had flu a month ago. He's looked grey since then and would lose his duster with me and would fall asleep in his chair after lunch which he never did before. He wouldn't consult the doctor during flu saying there was no need.

He complained about breathlessness for some time. I was at him for weeks to get to the doctor but you know what men are like — he didn't think it was bad enough.

Such conditions had been, to varying degrees, normalised without any action being taken. Sometimes, however, various remedies had been tried. Some men had been trying to cut down their weight or their smoking, on occasions with their doctor's advice. Others had been under treatment for a variety of conditions including indigestion and ulcers. One man, after treatment for arthritis, was described by his wife as

being determined to beat arthritis. He did strenous exercises for twenty minutes every morning. He also had what the doctor called dyspepsia every six months or so — it took him down to a shadow but he was never off work though he should have been. He's normally placid but the last two years he's been prickly, touchy and takes an hour or so to unwind in the evening — we have to keep out of his way then.

Another man had been attending a clinic every three months since hospital treatment for high blood pressure three years previously. His wife explained

About four or five weeks ago he wasn't feeling well and I suggested the doctor but he was due at the clinic soon so he thought they would check him, but they just said 'You're just the same — you haven't lost a pound — come back in three months.' It's maybe his weight but the clinic never really told him to get it down drastically.

Delay in Seeking Help

The decision to seek medical advice is determined by many factors: the symptoms, the severity and their perceived salience; the resulting disruption to work, family and other social activities; the frequency and persistence of the symptoms; the tolerance of the patient and family members; other competing needs and desires; the knowledge of services and their availability at that particular moment and the existing doctor-patient relationship. The initial mildness of symptoms may be the most potent cause of delay. From our series there is considerable evidence that most patients with mild and transitory symptoms initially prescribed delay for themselves : 'it's just an ache — it will pass off.' They hoped that the unpleasant and possibly threatening symptoms would go away and were encouraged in these hopes by previous health experiences. 'He said the pain was like a horse sitting on his chest', explained one woman, 'but when it was over he didn't see a need for going to the doctor. "If it happens again, I'll go", he said. Men *are* difficult.'

We wondered if current competing needs, such as the illness of a family member, had assumed priority and encouraged delay. In a few cases, specific events, sometimes unexpected such as an emergency operation to a family member, or sometimes already planned, such as the celebration of a family anniversary, had intervened between early and acute stages and probably delayed recognition of the latter. More often, however, the demands of normal social functioning, and particularly functioning in the occupational role, appeared to be accorded priority over earlier stages of discomfort or pain and often this process continued into the acute stage.

> On Monday after work he said he felt like a washed out cloth. He had a pain in his chest and arm but took some aspirin and went to work on Tuesday. He had a pain all Wednesday and had to keep stopping to get his breath even in the car. He was up all Wednesday night and I phoned from next door in the morning. He thought he had strained a muscle lifting at work two weeks ago.

In Chapter 5 we discuss some long-term, background pressures which may have predisposed these men habitually to ignore symptoms or make light of them and which we thought might also be relevant to their post-infarction careers. In the immediate pre-infarction career, the process of normalisation and delay in seeking help seemed to be two sides of the same coin.

Their husbands' resistance to entering the sick role was seen by
some wives as a characteristic of men in general; more often, it was
seen as a personality characteristic peculiar to their husbands. Sometimes, where doctors had previously labelled symptoms as minor,
wives emphasised that this had increased reluctance:

For longer than a year he's been tired and troubled with pain. I
had been on at him for a while to go to the doctor but since, before,
the doctor had always said it was just indigestion, or imagination,
he wouldn't go. I made an appointment for him but he got worse
before the day and I had to hurry it up. He wouldn't let me call the
doctor to him.

For most of these men, being eventually forced to 'give in' and adopt
the role of a help-seeker (and thus, presumably, an expressive role)
seemed to involve violating the norms by which they had previously
been able to conduct their lives and relationships — the norm of
fulfilling the demands of instrumental, particularly occupational, roles
at all costs; the norm of not fussing or worrying other family members;
and the norm of 'not wasting the doctor's time' with complaints that
might be considered trivial or temporary.

We looked for any evidence as to whether families with experience
of sudden heart illness in relatives acted more swiftly than others but,
although there were a few instances of very rapid identification and
action attributed to this, there were other instances where quick
action was taken by people with no previous experience while some
hesitated longer despite a family history. Nor could any consistent
differences between social class or age be detected in this respect.

Acute Onset

A considerable number of men carried on with their normal
activities, often despite quite severe pain, for instance completing
their day's work or their shift, finishing the shopping trip or driving
a family member to work. The abnormal symptom was pushed into
the background and the attempt was made to assert the normality
of things by continuing as if the symptoms were not there.

Sometimes, symptoms were explained by reference to a known
condition — indigestion or ulcer pain — and the remedies specific for
these conditions were applied. Where specific remedies were not
considered applicable, simple traditional remedies for minor health
problems were tried — a rest or sleep, something to drink, a walk in

the fresh air. One man, who developed pain while out for his usual evening walk with the dog continued to the pub as usual and had his accustomed two beers but added three whiskies — a combination of continuing normal activities and trying normal remedies.

Occasionally, a symptom, or degree of severity, was recognised as new and as requiring medical attention but the degree of urgency was not recognised so that appointments with general practitioners were made for two or three days ahead. In this group, it sometimes subsequently became necessary to summon emergency help before the appointment. A few visited doctors where labels such as indigestion or 'flu' were attached and simple treatment and rest prescribed. When after several days the normal and expected recovery did not take place or further more obvious symptoms appeared, rediagnosis by the family doctor or hospital admission produced the definitive diagnosis.

For most patients, however, the infarction itself was a traumatic event not easily forgotten by the man himself, or those with him (Table 4.2). He often experienced severe pain, a sense of impending death and powerlessness to control events. For a few men, there was a period ranging for several hours to days of which they had little memory. Some circumstances seemed to increase intensity of feelings. Among the few people who were engaged in physical exertion, the collapse was clear-cut and dramatic: this included men cutting down a tree, mixing concrete, dancing or moving furniture. Similarly, those who had collapsed in the street or in a hotel seemed to feel more deeply about public concern over their condition. One man was driving a car and another riding a bicycle when the pain developed.

Those who were alone, approximately one in five, often experienced feelings of great fear and helplessness. This particularly affected a man who was repairing his car at the weekend in the garage where he was employed. He had to open heavy sliding doors which presented considerable difficulty and took a long time; then, after partially recovering, he drove himself to his wife's work-place. Several men drove themselves either to the surgery or to the hospital casualty department, one in the middle of the night. One man who developed severe pain while driving alone in town, parked his car and went to his nearby solicitor's office, where help was summoned. Most men, however, were in a position where help could easily be obtained, seven out of every ten being in the company of a member of the family and more than half in their own homes, while a few became ill at work. Altogether, two thirds were seen by their family doctor before admission to hospital. In several instances a wife, son or friend drove men to their family doctor or to hospital, the latter more frequently occuring outside consulting hours.

Overall, in two out of every three cases wives were instrumental in summoning help, generally by telephoning from home or going to the nearest telephone. Occasionally a son or daughter was involved in the process. One woman said, 'If my daughter had not been there, I might have hung on till morning rather than leave him alone.' They had just arrived at a holiday cottage with no telephone and were ignorant of local medical services but their daughter's experience of working in a firm making cardiac care equipment encouraged her to seek aid quickly. No relatives other than children were involved but, where wives were absent or men at work, neighbours, business associates and factory nurses or first aiders sometimes summoned help.

A trained workmate, recognised as possessing more knowledge than family members, yet who is free from the inhibiting formalities which are seen as associated with approach to the medical profession, can be particularly valuable for men who lack practice in articulating their needs especially when their symptoms are imprecise. The role of a factory first aider in legitimising her husband's illness, giving treatment and sending him to hospital was acknowledged by one woman who said:

> He complained of pains at night but we thought it was indigestion. I suggested hot water. He went to work as usual in the morning but as soon as he got there he discussed his symptoms with the first aid boy and, together, they thought it might be his heart. He wouldna have liked to go to the doctor unless he was precise about what was wrong. The first aid boy gave him oxygen, without which he might have been worse, and sent him to hospital.

Another woman explained that her husband's pain had passed off by the time that they reached hospital and, as he was very suntanned after a recent holiday while she was distraught with fright, he 'felt like a fraud' when the receptionist asked him doubtfully: 'Are *you* the patient?' This illustrates how the 'extra burden of explanation', which E.J. Thomas[8] has described, may weigh on the disabled especially when there is no outward sign of illness. This extra burden may have also been a reinforcing feature in the marked resistance shown by a few men to some unacceptable aspect of the referral process. One man who became ill when some hundred miles from home rejected the local doctor's firm recommendation of immediate hospitalisation and insisted on a colleague driving him home. One refused to go to hospital until the visiting hour was over and another would not accept the doctor's offer of an ambulance for the journey to the hospital and insisted on travelling by bus.

Altogether, in this series (Table 4.3), nearly one third were admitted to hospital within one hour of the onset and recognition of the acute attack; half were admitted within two hours and three quarters within five hours. For approximately one in eight there was more than 24 hours delay before admission and, here, many factors contributed towards patient delay in seeking, or accepting medical advice. These final admission times compare favourably with findings in a study in Edinburgh in 1967, when the median time from the onset of the acute attack to arrival in hospital was 5 hours 23 minutes.[9] The difference could reflect the increasing realisation over the last few years among medical services that most deaths from myocardial infarction occur in the first few hours and that, with speedy response by medical and ambulance services, some are preventable; it may also partially indicate a geographical factor in the relatively compact nature of the smaller city.

In contrast, then, to popular belief but in accord with the impressions which we had gained from pilot interviews and previous experience, we found that the immediate pre-infarction career presented a very complex picture in which many men and their families appeared to have been normalising symptoms over a considerable period. We were particularly struck by the reluctance of so many to seek help, expressed by wives in such phrases as 'he wouldn't let me call the doctor', 'he wouldna have liked to go to the doctor unless he was precise about what was wrong', 'He felt it wasna anything to bother the doctor with'. Such attitudes seemed to be deeply embedded in a complex process of interaction between the patients' personalities and their social situations in which poor communication with medical services was a recurring feature.

A minority, however, did not show such attitudes. We thought that an explanation of the differences might be found partly in social networks surrounding patients which would act as 'lay referral systems' encouraging or discouraging the referral of their problems to medical services. Another part of the explanation might well lie deeper, reflecting the diverse types of socialisation processes to which patients and their wives had been exposed in childhood. Our intention was to look for differences between families in these and in other respects. Since many of the questions that we wanted to ask could not have been made meaningful for patients recovering from a different illness, we were unable to use external controls for this series. Instead, experience in pilot studies had convinced us that we should consider families as providing controls for each other in terms both of socio-demographic data and more subjective criteria.

In the next two chapters we discuss some of the background data which was obtained from wives during husbands' hospitalisation and which we thought might throw some light on the different ways in which men reacted to contingencies in the post-infarction career and which might also help to explain the different outcomes which they would reach.

Notes

1. Wadsworth, M. (1968). Planning with the Consumer in Mind. In: McKenzie, J. (ed.). *The Consumer and The Health Service,* London, Office of Health Economics.
2. Short, D. and Stowers, M. (1972). Earliest Symptoms of Coronary Heart Disease and Their Recognition. *British Medical Journal* 2, 387-91.
3. Yu, P.N. (1973). Pre-infarction Syndrome. In: Corday, E., and Swan, H.J.C. (eds.). *Myocardial Infarction,* Baltimore, The Williams and Wilkins Co.
4. Nixon, P.G.F. (1973). Coronary Heart Disease and Its Emergencies. *The Practitioner* 211, 5-16.
5. Mechanic, D. (1968). *Medical Sociology,* New York, The Free Press, p.122.
6. Robinson, D. (1971). *The Process of Becoming Ill,* London, Routledge and Kegan Paul.
7. Yarrow, M.R. *et al.* (1955). The Psychological Meaning of Mental Illness in the Family. *Journal of Social Issues* 11, 12-24.
8. Thomas, E.J. (1970). Problems of Disability from the Perspective of Role Theory. In: Glasser, P.H. and Glasser, L.N. (eds.), *Families in Crisis,* New York, Harper and Row.
9. Armstrong, A. *et al.* (1972). Natural History of Acute Coronary Attacks. A Community Study. *British Heart Journal* 34, 67-88.

5 PRE-CRISIS LIVING PATTERNS : THE LAUNCHING-PAD PHASE IN THE FAMILY LIFE CYCLE

The previous chapter has located the patients in the context of their pre-infarction health careers. In this chapter we seek to relate them to their setting in their occupational careers and within the family and community. We also begin to explore differences between families in respect of social factors which might influence response to contingencies in the post-infarction career and possibly outcome itself. This means considering socio-demographic data such as occupational roles as well as information on the health of other family members and indications of the kind of practical and emotional support available from informal social networks. It also entails an attempt to assess the presence or absence of life-change-events and ongoing difficulties which may have caused stress in the family before infarction and which may still be operative, engendering needs which compete with husbands' health needs. Here, the stage which families have reached in their life cycle and the confluence of major events demanding role change, such as death of parents, marriage of children, birth of grandchildren, may all be important in supporting or impeding the adjustments required after the illness.

Work Roles and Social Class

The meaning of work in relation to the recovery of heart patients is still a subject for controversy. Croog *et al.*[1] have pointed out that 'if work is actually a factor contributory to the occurrence of cardiac disability, its role in rehabilitation is a negative one'. Use of the concept 'definition of the situation' enables one to suggest as a corollary that if a factor such as work is *thought* to be contributory, then its role in rehabilitation may also be negative.

As indicated in the previous chapter, pre-infarction symptoms did not appreciably interfere with occupational functioning until the acute stage; consequently, at the time of infarction (Table 5.1), nearly all were currently of employed status, only four men being unemployed and another off work because of illness; this despite the fact that one in four subsequently defined themselves as having been ill at the time. Enquiry into stability of employment showed that over half had a stable record over the previous five years and only three men had experienced frequent changes. There was, however, evidence of some current disturbance or dissatisfaction in occupational roles, half the men claiming that they had been experiencing difficulty in coping, some expressing this in terms of physical condition and others in psychological terms. Further details and fuller description of the types of work involved are noted in Chapter 8 when they can be related to post-infarction modifications.

Social class was measured by the men's occupation at time of infarction, using the Registrar General's Classification. For most purposes, because of small numbers, the few clerical and sales workers in Social Class IIIa have been grouped with Social Classes I and II as 'Non-manual', while skilled manual workers in Social Class IIIb have been combined with semi- and unskilled workers (subsequently described as 'less skilled') in IV and V as 'Manual'. This is generally accepted as the most useful dichotomy to make since health and social indices suggest that the life-styles of persons in non-manual occupations in Social Class IIIa approximate more closely to those in Classes I and II than to those in the remainder of III but, where there are marked differences within the two broad groupings, these have been indicated. On this basis, the occupations of 28 men (21 in Classes I and II and 7 in Class IIIa) were classified as non-manual, and 48 (32 in Class III and 16 in Classes IV and V) as manual (Table 5.2).

As already indicated in Chapter 2, coronary heart disease is no longer necessarily associated with upper social class and the change is reflected in the distribution in this series. The recent appearance in national statistics of a positive gradient (i.e. increasing mortality in lower classes) among younger males is of particular relevance since younger manual workers are relatively frequently represented in this series, as shown in Table 5.2. In general, it might be expected that non-manual men would experience fewer difficulties in recovery, particularly since work might be more suitable or more easy to modify while greater financial resources could facilitate improved diets, for instance. Such differences, however, may be offset by other variables *within* social class groupings and it was part of the purpose of the study to take into account a number of other social characteristics.

Setting in Family and Community

Two out of every three families lived in a council house; this is not an unduly high figure for Scotland where a higher proportion of housing

is provided by local authorities than is the case in England (Table 5.3).
The fact, however, that over half the non-manual families lived in
council houses or privately rented property, while a few manual
workers owned or were buying their houses demonstrates something
of the overlap between social class groupings. Three out of four owned
either a car, or occasionally a motor cycle, and just under half had a
telephone (Tables 5.4, 5.5). Again these figures do not correspond
necessarily with social class, some non-manual families having neither
and some manual families both.

All except twelve couples were resident in the city, including
suburbs. The remainder lived in the countryside around or in small
towns. Stability in housing was high, one in every two families having
been living in the same house for over a decade and less than one in
five having moved in the two years preceding infarction. Further back,
however, there had been a fairly high degree of migration, nearly one
third of the men and well over one third of the women having been
born outside the area in which they were living (Table 5.6). Although
most of these incomers were married to each other, some were
married to sedentes, so just under half of all families included either
a husband or wife born elsewhere. Most of these came from rural areas
in neighbouring counties, but six men and eleven wives came from
other parts of Scotland, and four men and six wives from outside
Scotland; many had met their partners through work situations
especially service in the Armed Forces in the war years, but nearly
all had been living locally for two decades or more. Religious
affiliation also appeared stable, nearly nine out of every ten women
describing themselves as still belonging to the church or denomination
in which they had been brought up, others having changed to their
husband's faith or none; husbands were reported to be largely of a
similar distribution, all except twelve having been brought up in the
same denomination as their wives, and a few having changed to their
wife's faith or none (Table 5.7). Although a minority of families
derived great support from religious affiliation during the crisis and
recovery, this did not appear to be perceived as a particularly relevant
factor by the majority. Both migration status and religious denomination were considered as variables which might affect recovery but
neither appeared to show any association with outcome.

There were some indications (noted in more detail in Tables 5.8-
5.10) that a rather high proportion of men in this series (in non-manual
as well as in manual occupations) might have been exposed to social or
emotional disadvantage in childhood. Although the differences are not

large they appear rather more often than populations of comparable ages described in other studies[2,3] to have experienced less skilled parental occupation, early parental death and/or large family size. This might engender, consciously or unconsciously, a feeling of being 'relatively deprived', in the sense suggested by Stouffer[4], when comparing themselves with others seen as having experienced an easier upbringing — whether workmates, neighbours or perhaps their own children. Moreover, although wives also appeared somewhat disadvantaged in these respects in relation to the general population, the differences were slightly less than the men's in parental death and in family size. This may to some extent merely reflect the fact that men, being normally older than their wives, are slightly less likely to have benefitted from improved social conditions during their childhood. Never the less it may also suggest that this series of men may have been rather more restricted in the social experience of their upbringing and thus might also be susceptible to a sense of 'relative deprivation' in comparison with their wives, whose own social experience in upbringing would be a little more consistent with conditions in current family life-styles.

Social Networks as Resources

A main focus for this study was the extent and type of practical help and emotional support received from social networks and the use of networks as lay referral systems. Of particular interest was the part played by members of the families of origin of both spouses. The extent to which it is possible to receive help from kin is, of course, limited by their availability. This, in turn, is largely linked with age and migration, although not always consistently because, as was found in a migration study of a comparable area, Aberdeen,[5] some individuals (especially short-distance incomers from rural areas) had arrived in the area as young persons with their families of origin, while, in a few contrasting cases, sedentes were the only remaining representatives of their families of origin, all the others having died or left the area.

Local availability was defined as living at a distance from which a visit and return could be made within four hours, using whatever method of transport was habitual. If one accepts the presence of either father, mother or at least one sibling within this distance as constituting locally available kin, then, in their own right about one third of the men lacked any of these and so did a similar number of the wives (Table 5.11). However, four out of every five couples had at least one kin member available in respect of one spouse. This is, of course, a narrow definition of kin, and, in a few cases, cousins and aunts substituted in practice for closer kin, and, although excluded above, have been included later, where appropriate, as helpers or consultants.

Although many recent studies draw attention to the strength of the tie between married women and their mothers, they do not always show how much this pattern may be reinforced by age differences, especially as couples grow older. Since men are usually older than their wives, they are less likely to have parents alive than are their wives. For the same reason, reinforced by the fact that men die younger, among the parents of both spouses, mothers are likely to predominate. In this series (as already noted in Table 5.9), fewer than one quarter of the men had mothers living locally compared with over one third of the women, the corresponding figures for fathers being considerably lower. Among the minority, where parents were alive but outside the area, there was a similar pattern in which husbands' fathers were least often alive and wives' mothers most often, although the proportions were all lower. In only one family was a parent (a wife's mother) living in the household. Position in and size of the family can also affect availability of kin, the youngest member of a large family being not only less likely to have parents alive, but also less likely to have siblings alive compared with an eldest child.

We were particularly interested in the role of adult children as potential helpers (Table 5.12). Five married couples were childless and eleven others had children under sixteen years of age only. Two cohabiting couples, who were included on the grounds that the women were fulfilling the role of wife (and had been recognised in hospital records as next of kin), were childless in respect of their current households. The remaining fifty-eight families, just over three in every four, however, had at least one child of sixteen or over and, in nearly all of these, at least one child was residing at home or locally, so most families had the possibility of help from adult children as an alternative, or supplement, to members of their families of origin or to non-kin. In this respect they differed from the families studied by Bott[6] and McKinlay[7] who were at earlier stages in the family life cycle.

We had thought of trying to classify families along the lines suggested by Bott, i.e. distinguishing between families with joint marital roles and loose-knit networks on the one hand and segregated marital roles and close-knit networks on the other. As Bott[8] acknowledged however, although the extremes are easy to recognise, there are many intermediate and transitional couples and it is difficult to draw any clear cut dividing lines. Moreover, even the extremes were, in this series, by no means the most extreme possible. There were hardly any families whose networks could be positively classified as loose-knit; some incomers had merged into close-knit communities and the very few men who came near to the coronary stereotype of top executive were 'burgesses' with local orientations rather than 'cosmopolitans' or 'spiralists'; while at the other end of the scale very few workers were in traditional heavy industries where segregated roles are most usually found.

We found it possible, however, to make some distinction in terms of the persons from whom women acknowledged expecting and receiving help and support during the crisis and during the first year of the post-infarction career. These persons could be classified according to whether they were: children; members of wife's family of origin; members of husband's family of origin; non-kin; and, except in respect of help at the crisis, husbands. The categories of persons named and the number of different sources named could then be compared. To avoid repetition, some qualitative evidence of support, or lack of support, emanating from networks is discussed in Chapters 6 and 11, while in Chapter 12, wives' patterns of lay help and consultation are discussed in quantitative terms and some reasons for their association with outcome are suggested.

Wives' Work Roles

Two thirds of the women normally worked full-time or part-time, although five manual workers' wives were unemployed and one was on sick insurance at the time of husband's hospitalisation (Table 5.13). The proportion working varied with social class; half the women married to non-manual men were full-time housewives, one quarter were working full-time and one quarter part-time. Among manual wives only one quarter were not working or seeking work while two out of every five normally worked full-time and one third part-time.

Although the proportion of working wives appears high, this is not unduly high for this city and for this age group, particularly since it includes a substantial number of part-time workers. Dundee has, until recently, experienced a much higher level of female employment than any other Scottish city. Before marriage, one third of the women in this series had been in professional, technical or clerical work, one third had been divided between work in distributive trades (mostly as shop assistants), and skilled manual work; and the remaining one third had been in semi- or unskilled work.

There were no indications that wives going out to work might have been detrimental to their husbands' welfare. Housekeeping standards appeared high, although some of the full-time workers operated on very tight timetables, as a consequence of which, in some cases, it was only by arranging to drive them to hospital before visiting hours that time for interviews could be found. Few anticipated difficulties over their work roles when husbands first came home, some planning to take holidays or time off and others arranging for family members or kin to come in while they were out. (A policy of keeping patients at home from the beginning of the post-infarction career would, however, have presented more difficulties, partly because of the longer period involved and partly because of the suddenness.) Most working wives emphasised that having a second income gave a sense of security during their husbands' illness and, where husbands had previously been defined as suffering from serious illnesses, this had sometimes been a reason for wives taking on outside work or more work. Where manual workers' wives were unemployed, their inability to find work was often a source of worry and in some cases appeared related to their own poor health.

Wives' Health

At first interview two out of every three women reported having consulted a doctor in respect of some condition other than colds or very minor complaints during the year preceding husband's infarction; one in every ten claimed to have had some illness for which they had not sought medical advice and one quarter said that they had not been ill, apart from colds and very minor complaints (Table 5.14).

Half the women married to non-manual men reported consulting a doctor during the year compared with three quarters of manual wives. There was no consistent difference with wife's age at first interview, and little difference with husband's age, although wives of men in the oldest age group reported no illness slightly more often.

Women were also asked whether they had attended hospital as outpatient or inpatient during the preceding year. Ten women, or approximately one in every eight, had been admitted to hospital as inpatients, six of them for gynaecological operations, two for other operations and two for treatment for thyroid and 'nerves' respectively. Six other women attended hospital outpatient clinics for investigation or treatment. The remainder, who consulted general practitioners only, mentioned nervous conditions and menstrual troubles most frequently.

It is not suggested that the health record of these women was unusually bad but it was clear that many suffered from conditions likely to cause concern, and possibly stress, within the family both before and after infarction. Their ages ranged from a few in the late twenties to a few in the early sixties, one third being aged under forty-five and another third over fifty. The majority were therefore around menopausal age and many seemed to expect poor health for this reason. Never the less many of the conditions which they mentioned appeared to be of much longer standing and there was no evidence that the youngest or the oldest women had less health problems than the remainder. The indications pointed towards a long-term state of poor health rather than a build-up during the pre-infarction year but the existence of habitual health problems and the concern which they caused seemed likely to create a climate in which their husbands' symptoms might not always be accorded priority. As Rosenstock[9] has emphasised, illness behaviour takes place within a context where motives are frequently competing or in conflict.

Life-Change Events and On-going Difficulties

Apart from wives' health it seemed likely that some families might already, before the infarction, have been experiencing either a life-crisis or a long-term on-going difficulty in some 'area' which might either 'cause stress' or, at least, leave less 'room for manoeuvre' to the family in its adaption to the post-infarction career. It was recognised that concepts relating to stress are imprecise and controversial but it seemed worthwhile trying to assess, at first interview with wives, whether such difficulties existed and seemed likely to be still present as competing priorities for family concern during the post-infarction career.

The concept of 'areas' or 'domains' in one's life into which one can retreat at times of crisis has been used by Cohen and Taylor in *Psychological Survival*[10] with the implication that there is generally adequate 'room for manoeuvre' in these domains. Most disturbances, they write, 'are capable of resolution without profoundly affecting other parts of our life: we can pacify our wives, reassure our employers or avoid troublesome friends'. Even 'shattering' events, they continue, tend

> to occur in one part of one's life, in one domain. This means that the other domains can then be called into service to provide reassurance, to reestablish credibility. If one has to contend with the sudden loss of a close relative, then one can keep going by 'losing oneself in one's job'. Conversely the loss of employment can be compensated for by 'retreating into the family'. Sexual failures and tensions can (if sublimation theory is correct) be translated into artistic spheres, and sorrows can be muffled by drowning them in drink.

They go on to point out that long-term prisoners with whom they are concerned cannot play one domain off against another in this way, and, by implication, suggest that prisoners are unique in this respect. It seemed to us that persons in other situations of stress may also lack domains into which they can retreat. Furthermore, to suggest that domains can be played off against each other presupposes capacity for role flexibility. It also, by implying that other domains contain sources of strength to be drawn on at will, ignores the possibility that they may, on the contrary, already contain longterm difficulties which may deplete emotional resources or be likely to drain them in the future.

Our pilot studies had appeared to suggest that families with poor outcomes had started the post-infarction career with more difficulties than families with good outcomes. Those experiencing difficulties seemed more often to be manual than non-manual families and families with 'traditional' style marriages rather than those with 'partnership' marriages, although these two classifications did not always coincide.

It was decided to attempt independent assessment of 'areas of potential stress' to set beside a wife's definitions and expectations (which are considered in their own right in the next chapter) and to see how this related to outcome. The stress scale suggested by Rahe *et al.*[11] was considered but it seemed deficient, particularly in its omission of long-term life difficulties or on-going states. In particular, it omitted some kinds of possibly age-related stress which appeared important in this study. The most obvious examples were in respect of three families whose mentally handicapped children were in late adolescence or early adulthood; the possible stress associated with the condition at this stage seems

likely to be worse than in earlier years since on the one hand, there is
a sharper contrast when children of similar ages are becoming
independent while, on the other hand the parents are likely,
consciously or unconsciously, to be increasingly worried about the
children's future as they near retirement or death. It may be not so
much a *new* life event as the ageing of the family members which may
make it less easy to continue containing an earlier life event.

Another instance of stress possibly related to age seemed suggested
by the presence in a few families of considerably younger wives and of
'late' children — the gap between the age of husband and child
meaning that some men were playing the role of a father including
'rough and tumble' games (the likely continuance of which, during
recovery, caused apprehension to some wives), at an age when most
men are nearer the grandfather role.

Again, although Rahe's scale allows for the stress of a son or
daughter leaving home, events which are common to couples at this
stage of the family life cycle, it did not seem to cover some events
with long-term effects met in this series, such as a son suffering
permanent results of a serious accident (two families); sons in
trouble with the police, awaiting legal proceedings (two families —
although in both cases the boys were subsequently exonerated);
adult children encountering major marital difficulties (three families);
moreover, no provision is made on Rahe's scale for the possibility
that ageing may bring decreased ability to contain the same amount of
stress at work or in the family setting.

A further and more fundamental objection was that Rahe's scale
does not allow for variations in the meaning of stressful events for
different people. A number of writers have criticised his
quantitative approach on these grounds[12]. For such reasons,
although recent life event changes were recorded, no attempt was
made to quantify them in the way developed by Rahe and his
colleagues.

'Areas of Potential Stress'

Instead, the attempt was made to delineate five 'areas' or domains and
to assess, after first interviews, whether or not stress existed, and
appeared likely to continue during the post-infarction career, in respect
of any of these. In doing so, account was taken both of interpretations
implicit in the wife's expectations about husband's adjustment to the
post-infarction career and her definitions of his pre-infarction health.

This was supplemented by asking wives whether any troubles or changes in the nuclear family or families of origin (deaths, illness, weddings, births and other events which bring major role changes) had taken place in the year or two preceding the illness; probing was used to try to assess whether these events or effects proceeding from them were likely to be still operative in the post-infarction period. Wives were also asked about parents of both spouses and whether their health or living arrangements caused problems; and about their own health, work and commitments.

Probing was also used to try to assess whether problems mentioned by the wife, e.g. ill health of husband's mother, disagreements with neighbours, etc. were perceived by her as something that might worry her husband. Often, wives appeared to discount this, some saying 'I suppose it might' as though now admitting the possibility for the first time. One woman, referring to the discovery that one of their children was handicapped, recalled her doctor as explaining to her that her husband 'was even more upset than I was although he didn't show it', thus implicitly acknowledging that she had needed a professional interpretation before she could recognise her husband's concern. Some women, when asked why they thought that husbands had delayed mentioning symptoms, both before the illness and during the year following, gave replies such as: 'He mightn't want to worry me', thereby implying that there was already an area of concern focused on her health or her tendency to worry and that his symptoms had to reach a high level before they assumed priority over this.

Competing priorities such as these might make husbands disinclined to discuss problems with their wives and many were indeed said by their wives not to confide worries in them. Sometimes, there was evidence of the husband's illness having brought to the surface long-term anxieties previously unadmitted. One wife who said that she had been on pills for depression for a year attributed the depression to fear of cancer experienced since her husband's sister died of cancer five years previously; 'We were close to her and watched her going. I didn't think it worried him but he only told me last week [i.e. since his illness] that when I was ill two years ago he thought it was cancer but he didn't tell me.' (This wife also mentioned that one of their children, who had been attending the schools psychologist, was found to have excessive fears about death.)

After first interviews, wife's expectations on husband's adjustment and her interpretations on his personality, work situation and pre-infarction health were reviewed together with her answers to the questions outlined about on recent events and on-going difficulties in the nuclear family and network. From this review, assessment was made as to whether the family showed evidence of potential stress in one or more of five different areas. These were: (1) the existence of intercurrent illness of the husband other than the infarction itself; (2) difficulties likely to arise for the husband at work or in getting back to work; (3) difficulties relating to the husband's personality or the wife's perception of it; (4) difficulties in the nuclear family, e.g. health problems of wife or child, adolescent troubles of more than average seriousness; (5) difficulties in the network, e.g. excessively frail or demanding kin, or excessive disagreement with neighbours.

On this basis, half the non-manual families and two thirds of the manual families were assessed as containing three or more 'areas of potential stress' (Table 5.15). This is considered further in relation to outcome in Chapter 11.

It should be noted that where an area is assessed as containing potential stress, this may relate to two or more different conditions. For instance, in the nuclear family this might include wife's health as well as a problem with a child. In fact, many of the families for whom the largest numbers of areas of stress were assessed also contained more than one condition within each area.

It might be argued that the area of nuclear family should have been split into at least two sub-areas, one for the wife and one for children, but it was often difficult to distinguish, for instance, between stress arising primarily out of a condition relating to a child and that arising mainly from the woman's interpretation of that condition, so it seemed safer to group such conditions together.

Stage of Family Life Cycle: The Launching-Pad Phase

Although a few families were childless or had only very young children and a larger number had no children still living at home, the majority had some older children in the household and were, thus, at that stage of the family life cycle which is sometimes described as 'the launching-pad', a designation which implies a degree of tension and the need for preparation for role change and acceptance of moving into the 'post-parental stage'. At the same time, parents of both spouses were ageing and some deaths would be expected. The deaths were reported to have occurred during the preceding two years of five fathers and two mothers of husbands as well as one father and four mothers of wives. Several deaths of siblings and other close relatives were also mentioned and in some cases such deaths had involved husbands in considerable long-term worry and responsibility, clearing up family affairs, sometimes on behalf of the wife's family. In other families the health of parents was deteriorating.

Apart from bereavements which might generally be accepted as traumatic, attention has been drawn by Rahe and others to the potentially stressful effects of events which are generally expected to be entirely pleasurable. There seems some evidence in this series of such effects, both in respect of weddings of children and other relatives and in respect of celebration of the couples' own anniversaries. In one manual family with a large close-knit network the celebration of a twenty-fifth wedding anniversary immediately preceded the husband's heart attack. His wife described him as having been 'very wrought up'. The celebration had been planned for a long time, then there were difficulties over booking the hall and a lot of things 'going wrong'. It was suggested by one of their children that they should abandon the celebration but the husband insisted that it should continue. Finally, it was all arranged in a fortnight. This woman said 'You keep wondering whether it's going to go alright. We were both tensed up that night, wondering if the band was going to turn up. The money had all been arranged in advance but he could still have been worried.' At the second interview, she said: 'We can't think why it happened — he had no worries — people did wonder if it was our Silver Wedding, but he hadna been drinking and there was no trouble though I suppose it might have been excitement.' In another family, non-manual this time, the wife said that their daughter's wedding had been the only good thing amongst a number of troubles and family illnesses, adding: 'But there again, it can be a worry too because you want everything to go right.'

About half the families had one or more children living away from home at the time of first interview and most of these departures had involved marriages in the preceding few years. During the year following husband's illness, there were changes involving children in approximately half the families. Generally this meant a wedding or the birth of a grandchild and had been foreshadowed in the previous year. In more than one case, the husband was just home from hospital in time for a wedding planned before his illness. One family experienced the weddings of three children in the two years before the illness. In another family, one daughter was married in the year before the illness and one in the year following the illness. This wife said that her husband was 'broken hearted' over the younger one's marriage because he thought she was too young. In addition, the two weddings had been very expensive. She added, 'The children, especially the wee one,

wouldna see us wanting for anything, but you have to put a face on
it — they've just started their own married lives and they
have plenty of troubles of their own — it's not fair to put it
on them.'

There were other indications that wedding preparations involved
many families in a long drawn out process of negotiating role change,
which, especially where social experience was restricted and family
communication limited, might make excessive demands both on
economic and emotional resources. Such situations may be all the
more exhausting, because of the social norms prescribing cheerfulness
on such occasions and the taboo on showing worry, depression or
irritation.

We found ourselves in agreement with Parkes[13] that it is hard to
know whether a given life-event such as the marriage of a child is to
be construed as a gain or a loss. Moreover, although pre-wedding
rituals may once have had the effect of easing role change, the
apparently inexorable demands of contemporary commercialised
versions, when superimposed on everyday domestic routines, may
only increase stress. Sometimes, given the analogy of the launching-
pad, the further analogy of countdown seemed hardly too extreme
to convey the level of tension engendered.

Interpenetration of Events and Long-term Difficulties

Other life change events were more difficult to separate from
on-going states, and there was a good deal of evidence pointing to
interpenetration between them, suggesting the cumulative effect over
time of a number of events and states.

One man had changed within his profession to a more demanding
specialism about four years before his illness. His wife thought that,
ever since then, he had had difficulty in 'unwinding' each evening
when he came home from work. Then, three years before his illness
she had a bad road accident and was in hospital for some months and
incapacitated for a long time thereafter. She said, 'We were just getting
back to normal when this happened.' There had also been worry about
the husband's mother's health and the breakup of a daughter's
marriage; finally the youngest child had an emergency operation just
before the husband's illness.

Another woman, married to a manual worker, said that all their
friends and relatives ascribed her husband's illness to the effects of a
son's accident three years previously. This son had major and
permanent injuries, and the hospital had given them no hope for

survival for the first few weeks. Although he had recovered and was working, her husband still worried constantly lest his injuries damage his prospects both in employment and in marriage.

In another manual family, one adult son had died suddenly from a heart condition three years previously, while a teenage son, whom his mother described as 'unfortunate' had experienced, from infancy onwards a history of sudden illness and accidents, including one shortly before her husband's illness. 'The lad's always been a worry', she said, 'and in accidents all his life — whenever I see anyone in a white coat or an ambulance I always think it's for him.'

In other families, events which were seen in themselves as minor, when coupled with long-term difficulties, appeared to have built up to a cumulative or additive effect. For instance, a shopkeeper's wife with an adult handicapped child explained

> There've been a lot of little things lately — the shop is liable to be taken over for redevelopment and compensation will be poor. And there was a break-in a few months ago and we had a shock about that, having to clear up the mess. Then the lights failed the week before my husband's illness and he had to rush round looking for an electrician and couldn't find one.

They had also been helping elderly relatives to move house, undertaking on their behalf a programme of cleaning, laying carpets and decorating in evenings and weekends.

A manual worker's wife said that her mother had died two years previously. Both their children had married during the two years following, and one was now awaiting a divorce. This wife, who herself was awaiting admission to hospital for an operation, had been hospitalised on account of a nervous breakdown four years previously.

Sometimes, on-going states were seen as improvements; a nightwatchman's wife felt that the year previous to her husband's illness had been a better one in many ways than the preceding ones. He had accepted a demotion from a more responsible job because this had involved much travelling, so that he could get home every day. She said, 'In a way it was the happiest year — then there was a rumour of redundancy for six weeks — then one week's notice — and he had a month off work before his illness began.' There had also been trouble for a few years with neighbours whom she described as a rough, noisy crowd in the flat above and it seemed likely that her husband had been anxious not to leave her alone so much. Although they had been in the city for many years they were still very conscious of their incomer status from a rural background.

In only one family did a wife directly attribute the cause of her husband's illness to a family quarrel. She described her husband as very strong willed and their sons as having always disliked his heavy drinking habits. Then one son took a job in the same work place as his father and took the opposite side in a union dispute. This led to a bitter quarrel about three or four months before the illness and the son had been thinking of emigrating. This woman observed: 'Some people bring illness on themselves — sometimes it seems like a judgement of God but you love them all the same, even though you think they're wrong.'

Other less dramatic life change events commonly encountered at this stage in family life were described in terms that did not suggest unduly emotional reactions. Never the less, since many husbands were described as playing down physical ailments and being reluctant to communicate worry, one might expect that their difficulties in adjusting to problems associated with children maturing and leaving home may also be greater than they, or their families, acknowledge. Qualifications or reservations made by women suggest that some such process may be in operation — for instance in one family where the wife said: 'We've had no *real* trouble, except our daughter wants to marry before her fiancé finishes college, but we wouldn't make an issue of that'; and in another family: 'Its only that our daughter's marrying someone in a different faith and you always want more for them than you had yourself.' Implicitly these women were revealing their doubts although hardly liking to articulate them and it seemed likely that acknowledging this would be even more difficult for the husbands.

Children's departure was not always directly associated with a recent marriage but might still be stressful for some parents. One woman described her husband as having been depressed since their only son had emigrated several months previously: they had been planning to visit him on holiday so that they could find out whether they should go and settle near him. In another family, both children had left home at the same time a few months before their father's illness — one to work in England after being made redundant locally, one to join her husband abroad.

It seemed that life change events and on-going states, even when not explicitly recognised as particularly stressful, were presenting problems requiring role change and adjustment which, for many families, seemed unresolved and often only partially recognised at the time of infarction. Coupled with difficulties or threats in the work situation they seemed to promise an uneasy background against which the role changes required in the post-infarction career would have to compete.

Apart from some overt health problems in which, as we have seen, general practitioners were sometimes involved, and occasional contact with educational services over children, such troubles were seen as something to be endured and contained within the family, and not as anything for which professional help might be sought. It could, of course, be argued that such events and states amount to no more than is normal for this stage in the family life cycle. Never the less, some families in this series appeared to be more heavily weighed down in these respects than were others and, to this extent, some men appeared to be starting out on their post-infarction career already at a considerable disadvantage.

Notes

1. Croog, S.H., Levine, S. and Lurie, Z. (1968). The Heart Patient and the Recovery Process : A Review of the Directions of Research on Social and Psychological Factors. *Social Science and Medicine* 2, 111-64.
2. Illsley, R. and Thompson, B. (1961). Women from Broken Homes. *Sociological Review* 9, 27-54.
3. Young, M. and Willmott, P. (1957). *Family and Kinship in East London,* London, Routledge and Kegan Paul.
4. Stouffer, S.A. (1949). *The American Soldier.* Princeton, N.J., Princeton University Press.
5. Illsley, R., Finlayson, A. and Thompson, B. (1963). The Motivation and Characteristics of Internal Migrants. *Milbank Memorial Fund Quarterly* XLI, 2, pp.115-43. and 3, pp.217-48, New York. Reprinted in Jansen, C.J. (ed.) *Readings in the Sociology of Migration* (1970) Oxford, Pergamon, pp.123-56.
6. Bott, E. (1957). *Family and Social Network: Roles, Norms, External Relationships in Ordinary Families,* London, Tavistock.
7. McKinlay, J. (1973). Social Networks and Utilization Behavior, *Social Forces* 51, 275-92.
8. Bott, E. (1971). *Family and Social Network: Roles, Norms and External Relationships in Ordinary Urban Families. Reconsiderations,* 2nd edn., London, Tavistock.
9. Rosenstock, I.M. (1960). What Research in Motivation Suggests for Public Health. *American Journal of Public Health* 50, 295-302.
10. Cohen, S. and Taylor, L. (1972). *Psychological Survival,* Harmondsworth, Penguin, pp.42-3.
11. Rahe, R.H., Meyer, M., Smith, M., Kjaer, G. and Holmes, T.H. (1964). Social Stress and Illness Onset. *Journal of Psychosomatic Research* 8, 35-44.
12. Hinkle, L.E. (1972). The Concept of 'Stress' in the Biological and Social Sciences. *Paper Presented at the Third International Conference on Social Science and Medicine,* Elsinore. (Mimeographed).
13. Parkes, C.M. (1972). *Bereavement,* London, Tavistock.

6 PROBLEMS AND RESOURCES: WIVES' EXPECTATIONS AND DOUBTS

As already explained the experience of pilot interviews shaped our approach to the main series. In particular, this suggested that to use the concept of 'definition of the situation' fruitfully in the context of the post-infarction career, it should be stretched to include expectations and interpretations of specific problems. Wives in the pilot study had said at one extreme, 'I didn't really worry because I knew he would be sensible and they would be understanding at work', and at the other extreme, 'I was sure he wouldn't be able to stop smoking and that the job would be too much for him.' We wanted to find, in the main series, whether such expectations and interpretations were present from the beginning and whether they were associated with social characteristics of the families and with outcome.

A number of studies have suggested that expectations of significant others about the recovery of a patient may be self-fulfilling. For instance, Freeman and Simmons[1] have shown that former mentally ill patients returning to conjugal homes exhibit higher performance levels than those returning to parental homes; they hypothesise that expectations may be higher in conjugal homes and patients may rise to meet the challenge.

The career concept facilitated consideration of the effects of past social experience on the pathways likely to be followed. Drawing on Lemert's[2] use of this concept in terms of typical or recurrent contingencies and problems awaiting patients, experience in the pilot interviews suggested that those concerned with wives' perception of the work situation, exercise, smoking, money and consulting doctors would be the most fruitful in that they appeared to be regarded as very important by wives.

Wives were interviewed (generally at home, occasionally at their place of work or in the interviewer's car,) while husbands were in hospital. It was not possible to standardise the time after infarction with any precision but it was always between five and twenty days and generally around the second week.

Degree of severity was not known at the time of first interviews with wives and it seemed an advantage to be working 'blind' in this respect. The women had all just passed through a crisis in which they

were aware that their husbands might have died. They laid considerable
emphasis on their husbands' continued survival being seen as
conditional — '*If* he does as he's told', '*If* he's careful'. Their major
concern was with defining the practical implications for the future —
how the restrictions seen as imposed, both by the illness itself and the
conditional nature of recovery, could be fitted in with their husbands'
usual way of living, particularly in respect of his work situation but
also taking into account his personality, interests and social commitments. This concern was common to all, differences appearing in the
degree to which they expected that husbands would or could comply,
and in the particular areas (work situation, personality, smoking, diet,
etc.) which many foresaw as hindering or threatening this compliance.
Such role rearrangements as they anticipated for themselves were
contained within the framework of adjustments which they foresaw as
needed by their husbands.

Each woman was asked: whether she thought her husband's work
was suitable as it was and, if not, would he be able to adjust it, or
change it if necessary; whether he would be likely to adjust leisure
time activities, especially exercise and smoking; whether she thought
he would consult his doctor about any difficulties occurring during
recovery; whether money was likely to be a big problem; and what, if
any, difficulties she foresaw both for her husband and for herself.
Answers on five specific contingencies were coded into those where
she had favourable expectations, i.e. no problems were foreseen in
respect of this specific contingency — work, exercise, smoking,
consulting doctor, money; and those where she had unfavourable or
doubtful expectations. The two questions on general difficulties
foreseen for her husband and herself served to summarise and
recapitulate on the specific expectations and to allow her to define
more idiosyncratic problems; answers were similarly assessed as
favourable (i.e. no obstacles which the wife foresaw her husband or
herself being unable to cope with); or unfavourable (some or many
obstacles). Wives were encouraged to expand on their answers and as
much detailed comment as possible was noted. (Detail for the
following sections is given in Tables 6.1 and 6.2, based on eighty-eight
men, that is including twelve who died during the year before second
interview; as indicated in Chapter 1, detail on these twelve men is also
given separately in the Appendix).

Relative Infrequency of Favourable Expectations

In general, women were most worried over work and smoking,

approximately three out of every five anticipating difficulties in respect of each. These were not always the same women, some expressing concern about work only and others about smoking only.

Previous studies have suggested that work is often blamed by wives with the implication that this, consciously or unconsciously, serves to divert attention from the possible effect of domestic difficulties. However, such studies do not seem to have enquired whether wives who indict work expect this to remain a problem during the post-infarction career. In this series, as in the pilot interviews, wives who mentioned work or overwork as a cause did not appear worried if they also defined this as a temporary feature or one which they perceived as capable of being modified. Wives who were worried, however, drew attention to long-term factors either in the requirements of their husband's job or their attitude to work, or both. Sometimes these women defined the difficulties in terms of personality, 'the firm might be alright but *he* drives himself too hard' or 'its not the nature of the work — its *his* nature that's the trouble'. The converse definition in terms of external factors also appeared — 'He's sensible enough but, the way things are just now, *they* may not be able to make it easier for him' or 'He wouldn't mind changing but I don't see him being able to get a lighter job — there just aren't any': in the deteriorating local economic situation over the period of the study, such anxieties were expressed more frequently. Where either work or the husband's attitude to work, or both, were perceived as difficulties, wives seemed to see their husbands as trapped in a complex situation which they were unable to alter.

Although two out of every five women did not consider smoking to be a worry, this proportion was inflated by several who were married to lifelong non-smokers or, more usually, to men who had ceased smoking some years previously. When these are deducted, then only one quarter were confident that husbands would now abandon the habit. The initial response of some was to express confidence on the grounds that 'He *has* stopped now' (i.e. while in hospital), but on closer questioning, these wives often admitted that they doubted if this would continue, and only wives who appeared really confident that their husbands would not resume after leaving hospital were coded as having favourable expectations. Such women would generally add some reinforcement such as 'He has great willpower' or 'He's had such a fright — he's determined to stop', whereas those with negative or doubtful expectations would say 'I don't think he *can* stop' or 'It means such a lot to him — I don't know if he *can*.' (Wives' own smoking habits and intentions are discussed later in Chapter 9.)

Overall, while less than half the wives held favourable expectations on work and smoking, the other specific contingencies more often yielded favourable expectations. Over half the women did not anticipate money being a big problem during the illness and recovery period (it should be remembered that the interviews took place in the early 1970s, before inflation became a 'normal' worry), just under two thirds considered that husbands would consult general practitioners about any difficulties occuring during recovery and a slightly higher proportion thought that they would follow advice about leisure time activities, including taking moderate exercise. In answer to the latter question, most wives with unfavourable expectations defined their doubts in terms of husbands' personality, some doubting their ability to give up what were, in their view, over-strenuous leisure time activities, e.g. 'fanatical' car repairing for friends and acquaintances, while in contrast others feared inactivity and doubted their willingness to walk regularly, sometimes blaming this on car-owning. The relevance of pre-infarction illness was emphasised by a few women whose husbands had previous artery trouble which made walking difficult.

Women who were confident that husbands would consult doctors often explained this in terms of positive personality qualities, for instance, a baker's wife, 'He's so open about things like that'; a sales manager's wife, 'He likes to know what goes on'; a garage proprietor's wife, 'He's normally good at going to the doctor — he'd rather find out — I'm more inclined to put things off — *he* likes to know.' Other women who were also confident often referred to qualities in the doctor or the practice: a farmer's wife, 'The doctor is easy to talk to'; a ship plater's wife, 'They are good friends — the doctor is very understanding'; the wife of a previously disabled man in sheltered employment, 'The doctors here [in the practice] are more like friends of the family.'

In contrast, many women who were doubtful or who thought that their husbands were unlikely to consult their general practitioners explained this in terms of negative characteristics of their husbands, often adding references to their own roles in this context. A labourer's wife explained, 'He never would go — unless I was to force the issue'; a painter's wife, 'He's not good at asking, not one for pushing himself forward — sometimes he leaves it to me'; a supervisor's wife, 'Our doctor is very quiet and he's quiet too — I can chatter to doctors but he won't approach unless asked to'; a joiner's wife, 'I was surprised when he did go — I knew then he must be feeling bad — he's the sort of man who doesna like to worry you.'

Some women foresaw the possibility of change in attitudes to doctors because of the fright caused by the heart attack. A buyer's wife said 'He's been shaken — he has been reluctant in the past to see the doctor but he would be honest.' A bus driver's wife explained, 'He might talk to me and he might change now and talk to the doctor — formerly he wouldna have'; and a shopkeeper's wife said 'In the past he never felt ill *enough* — he had lots of aches and pains but he didn't feel he *should* go — now he'll be more aware that it is the correct thing to do.' Several suggested, however, that their own intervention might still be needed. A farm worker's wife said, 'I always have to be at him to go but it *may* be better now — still I'll maybe see the doctor first — I could tell him more than he would say'; a postman's wife, 'He isna keen on doctors really but I'll have to see the doctor and he'll have to get it to him (not to overdo it).'

In addition to the questions on the five specific contingencies, wives were asked if they saw 'in general' any or many difficulties for their husbands and if so what. This question, besides recapitulating on the specific expectations, also gave them an opportunity to bring out more idiosyncratic difficulties — for instance diet problems, which had not been specifically included because some of the men were not overweight and were not given diet advice (some of these are discussed in Chapter 10). It also gave them an opportunity, which many of them took, to make interpretations about husbands' psychological characteristics, similar phrases recurring very frequently — 'perfectionist', 'over-conscientious', 'He doesna tell you things', 'He keep things to himself', 'He tears like an idiot, if he were five minutes late that was no good', 'He's always hashing on as if there wasna to be another day.' In such phrases wives were often, explicitly or implicitly, attributing the cause of their husband's illness to such characteristics and defining them as permanent or difficult to alter and as detrimental to the post-infarction career. In all, only one third of the women expected no difficulties for their husbands.

Fewer still — only one in every four — anticipated no difficulties for themselves. Where wives anticipated difficulties for themselves, but not for their husbands, these were often in respect of their own role arrangements and most appeared confident that they could make practical adjustments fairly easily. Some working wives foresaw possible temporary difficulty over their own jobs or hours of work; wives of some self-employed men suggested that they would take a more active part in the business; a few women thought that they might take up driving again or learn to drive; many said that they and their children would take on some of the husband's household tasks such as decorating or gardening; a few with young families thought that they would have to manage with less help from their husbands over the children.

When women anticipated difficulties both for themselves and for their husbands and when they considered that these arose more from his own nature than from external sources, they tended to describe difficulties in such terms as — 'his thinking he can go on exactly as before' or 'his wanting to do too much too soon' and their own difficulties as — 'getting him to do what he's told'. One woman, when asked what difficulties she anticipated for herself, replied succinctly, 'Just my husband.'

Thus, overall, on two of the most important contingencies, work and smoking, less than half the wives had favourable expectations about their husbands' ability to adjust, and on no specific contingency was the proportion of wives with favourable expectations higher than 70 per cent. Moreover, only one third expected no difficulties 'in general' for their husbands and less than a quarter that there would be no difficulties for themselves. Many women with unfavourable expectations seemed resigned to the unlikelihood of anything, even the shock of the illness, changing their husband's way of life or his work situation in a long-term way. They did not seem to expect that anyone could help with either of these problems.

Differences between Families on Specific Expectations

The pilot interviews had suggested that there might be social class differences influencing both expectations and outcome, even although there might also be, within social class groupings, other factors cutting across, especially type of social network. Some differences in expectations between class and age groups are described here, and more detail is given in Tables 6.1 and 6.2. Some illustrations of the way in which wives perceived social networks as operating at the time of the crisis are also given here while an attempt to make a quantitative assessment of networks as coping resources is deferred until Chapter 12 when this can be related to outcome.

Differences between the wives of non-manual workers and skilled manual workers were not large in respect of expectations about work adjustment, but there was a considerable drop in expectations among wives of less skilled workers. Differences between classes disappeared in respect of expectations on exercise.

On smoking, however, the major difference occurs between wives of non-manual men, over half of whom held favourable expectations, compared with the wives of skilled manual men, less than one third of whom held favourable expectations, and the wives of less skilled workers, only just over one quarter of whom held favourable expectations. The gradient on expectations about money was much steeper and, here, there was less difference in the proportion of wives holding favourable expectations between non-manual wives and the wives of skilled manual workers but a very sharp drop occurred between the latter and the wives of less skilled workers.

So far, the class differences are not unexpected. An interesting anomaly, however, occured in respect of expectations on consulting doctors. Here, non-manual wives were, as would be expected, more confident than wives of either group of manual wives, but wives of less skilled workers appeared more confident than wives of skilled workers. This can be explained by the presence amongst the less skilled workers in this series (compared with the skilled men) of a higher proportion with pre-infarction histories of serious medical conditions (including blindness, amputation, major operations and previous cardiovascular troubles). Such men had accepted previous medical regimens and were already very dependent on their doctors so their wives knew that they would be ready to consult them, often describing the husband as being 'a good patient'. Both spouses were accustomed to making adjustments to the husband's previous illness or disability and their expectations of 'normal life' had already been lowered. This did not, however, necessarily prepare them for the more active role flexibility required by the new illness.

In this context it is also interesting to look at the divergence in expectations between the wives of non-manual and skilled manual wives. On several contingencies the difference was not great, but it was at its widest on the likelihood of husbands consulting doctors (over four out of five compared with under half). This would suggest that, while wives of skilled manual workers had expectations which came close to those of non-manual wives on some material issues, they were less confident in an area — the habit of consulting doctors — which is more conditioned by different class socialisation patterns in early childhood and is thus more resistant to change.

The wife of a van driver related how she had worked in a doctor's house as a young girl and had got used to their way of doing things but her husband's mother was very old fashioned and strict and 'didn't welcome doctors'. Her husband had told her that he had been taken into hospital at the age of seven for a tonsil operation, not having been warned about it in advance and thus 'he got a terrible shock — he's been afraid of hospitals and doctors ever since'. Consequently, when his wife urged him to go to the doctor he wouldn't give in for some days — 'until the pain was so bad — it wasn't bad enough until then'. She was doubtful whether even the shock of a heart attack would make him more ready to consult his doctor.

Among the small number of pilot interviews age had not emerged as influential but in the main series it began to assume importance. When all social classes were combined and broken into four age groups, wives of men in the two oldest groups held favourable expectations more often than wives of men below 50, and more especially below 45. Exceptions were in respect of money, where wives of both the younger age groups appeared more confident, and in respect of consulting doctors, where age seemed to make little difference. In general, the greater confidence of wives of older men may reflect their husbands' approach to retirement and possibly readier acceptance of adjustments required by ageing. Some of the wives, however, appeared to anticipate more difficulties for themselves, possibly implying that they were expecting to take on a more active role following their husbands' illness.

Indications of Differential Interpretations among Social Networks

In addition to the wives of manual workers having lower expectations, they also appeared more often to believe that nothing could be done to alter things or, alternatively, they seemed more often likely to handle attempts at role change in an inappropriate way. Phrases such as 'We'll all get on to him to stop smoking' suggested an aggressive approach which might well be counterproductive. In contrast, non-manual wives appeared more often confident that difficult role transformations could be achieved by joint endeavour and by means suited to their husbands' personalities. For instance, one, married to an older business man, explained, 'I won't rush him about retiring — I'll just let him come to it gradually himself'; and a supervisor's wife, recognising that her husband would pay more attention to the views of their daughter (who had a scientific qualification) said that she would leave the latter to persuade him to cut down on smoking.

A further advantage for non-manual families was that they more often appeared to have access to lay consultants with experience of recent coronary heart disease and so more often encountered definitions that were congruent with professional definitions. A woman, herself a teacher in a prosperous, close-knit community, said that many people had spoken to her about her husband's illness and all had been helpful. Some were people whom she said she hardly knew but they had never the less telephoned or stopped her in the street to give her the benefit of their experience, or the experience of acquaintances; thus she soon realised that many people in the community had experienced coronaries without her having ever known this. (Implicit in this is the suggestion that, having previously perceived these persons as 'normal', she could more easily accept that her husband would similarly 'return to normal'.) She considered all the advice that she had received as constructive, especially on exercise and diet. On the latter point, advice from medically qualified friends was particularly appreciated as she considered that given by the hospital was somewhat inadequate. However, she also made a point which demonstrates that networks, even if helpful after infarction, may yet fail to fulfil a preventive function. She said

> We had known lots of people who'd had this but they were all about ten years older. He wasn't old enough to think he was likely to have it. We know *now* that its quite common earlier. Also, he had an annual medical examination with the Forces until a few years ago and was always first class, so we thought there was no possibility of anything being wrong.

A businessman's wife whose husband was also in his forties made a similar point. She said 'I suppose we really are the age group which is just coming up to this trouble, rather than those who have been through it. Probably the normal person would be in the 50s to 60s age group. Anyone younger would be the exception rather than the rule.' These two examples illustrate how, even in circles where knowledge may be generally congruent with professional definitions, individuals may fail to identify themselves with an 'at risk' group, suggesting that even the best informed lay referral systems may be at present less valuable in prevention than in recovery.

Never the less, in all other respects, non-manual families seemed at an advantage in their readier access to reference groups possessing stocks of knowledge about successful outcomes with which they could easily identify as well as 'recipes for action' which they saw as realistic. They also appeared, by virtue of their occupations or reputations, to be more often protected against lack of congruence over advice. A young professional couple, both upwardly mobile in terms of their parents' occupations and living in a council house, appeared aware of the possibility of lack of congruence. This woman explained

> Knowing my husband, people would shy off giving advice. They know he would take the expert advice, not old wives' tales. It was the same with our children — my mother said 'do it your way' even though she has occasionally advised when I've asked her.

One non-manual family which was exposed to a diversity of definitions, some of them negative, ran a small shop and their customers were described as 'mostly telling cheerful stories but some tell the other kind'. This woman added that, when visiting her husband in hospital, she heard another visitor commenting adversely to him on his age and usual diet which, she felt, made her husband look anxious. It was after this that her husband had a second attack and she felt that the visitor's remarks had not helped. In this case the visitor and the husband were both incomers from the continent to the wife's community of origin and perhaps this made her particularly sensitive to the visitor's assumption that he was entitled to say something pessimistic to her husband, thus deviating from the norms which she and her family held.

In two other families, both manual ones, where wives expressed concern about 'sad tales', there was more than usual discontinuity between husband's network and wife's network. A woman who felt apart from the local community to which her husband belonged, and to which she was an incomer, quoted as one of her main worries 'Job's Comforters', adding 'its not so much *what* they say as *how* they say it — that he will have to be *so* careful'. She claimed to having stopped going out to avoid this during her husband's hospitalisation. Another woman, who was cohabiting with a man awaiting separation said,

> When you're waiting to visit, you hear people saying 'they'll never be the same again'. Well, I don't think that's right. I think he can be the same, but some of his visitors don't help. They all come in and all ask the same thing: 'Well how did it happen? And he has to talk or tell about it all the time. Yesterday, friends who hadn't been there before were visiting him so he had to go through it all over again. I could see beads of sweat on his brow, and I've been worried about it all day, but it wouldn't do to say anything.

These three examples are all cases where discontinuity in networks may have had the effect of making the wife unusually sensitive to negative interpretations, but the next few examples show that lack of congruence may also exist between different generations of close kin. A manual worker's wife who chose her daughter's mother-in-law as a consultant in preference to her own mother explained, 'My mother told me about someone she knew but I've got to the stage now where I don't listen to her. She tends to dwell on the gloomy side. She was offended because I went to speak to my daughter's mother-in-law first instead of going to her.' In this case, the daughter's mother-in-law was younger and was felt to be more up-to-date and knowledgeable.

Several women who described themselves as 'not one to listen to what other people say or to take secondhand advice', appeared to be defending themselves against the possibility of being told 'sad tales'. A former countrywoman contrasted the unhelpful attitude of older relatives with the way their son saw things:

> I wish people wouldn't say some things — my elder sister said on the phone 'maybe he'll take a shock now' and my son was in the room and he said, 'she oughtn't to say that' — of course they live in the country and are not used to things the way they are now. My husband's sister is also inclined to depress you a bit. She's not been so bad this time, but after his previous operation she said 'you're looking proper poorly', and my son said 'how tactless can you be?' I did tell her then and so she has been better about it this time. Its not so much depressing as annoying when people know more about your business than you do yourself. I think that they should wait for *you* to tell *them*.

Another tradesman's wife made it clear that she selected some definitions and rejected others:

> I lead such a busy life, I havena time to listen. A friend with a husband who had a heart attack said 'don't treat him as an invalid', and that's sensible. I think people could be depressing if you listen, but I'll stick to what the hospital doctor said. My aunt, who is 80, said, 'They're never the same again' — you can forgive her, being old, but I think its better to cut people off before they start telling you.

Where manual workers' wives did refer to reassuring definitions these often came from people outside the immediate circle of close friends and relatives, one who was herself in clerical employment, recounting that her boss had told her that he had had two attacks — 'It's been a help hearing how you get back to gradually doing more things.'

Occasionally, reassurance had been partly obtained from an entirely fortuitous encounter. A tradesman's wife explained

> It's mostly been helpful — when you get talking it doesn't seem so drastic — it's mostly people at work, and neighbours, who tell of people back at normal life, and even a lady down at the office where I went to see about my husband's car insurance — she sorted it all out and told me how her husband had a heart attack and lived quite normally, and also she pointed out their manager who had two attacks — it's not so drastic when you hear this.

Sometimes, neighbourhood figures of professional or paramedical standing — several nurses, a hospital technician and a chemist — were mentioned as sources of advice or of reassuring definitions but such occupations appeared to be very thinly represented in the majority of networks[3] and many manual families appeared unlikely to encounter any lay consultant whose experience would approach congruence with professional definitions.

Thus, even while the men were in hospital, it was possible to see from interviews with their wives that the expectations to which they would be exposed on returning home were (like the background situations described in the previous chapter) very diverse and appeared likely to place many of them, particularly some manual workers and younger men, at a considerable disadvantage. It seemed, indeed, appropriate to recall the derivation of the word 'career' from *carrière* — a race course. One began to see the post-infarction career in terms of a partially overgrown race course, its outer tracks invaded by bush: a few well-equipped runners were starting on relatively smooth inner tracks while the unprepared majority, already impeded by heavy burdens, would stumble over uneven ground beset with thorns and briars.

Notes

1. Freeman, H.E. and Simmons, O.G. (1958). Mental Patients in the Community: Family settings and performance levels. *American Sociological Review* 23, 147-54.

2. Lemert, E.M. (1961). *Human Deviance, Social Problems and Social Control*, New Jersey, Prentice Hall, p.50.
3. To avoid repetition the method used in classifying women's lay help and consultation networks both at hospitalisation and twelve months later is described in Chapter 12 together with their association with outcome.

  ACCEPTING – OR DOUBTING – NEW
DEFINITIONS IN HOSPITAL AND HOME

The social space created by emergency hospitalisation is a vacuum into which new definitions rush. Initially the varying degrees of physical pain or discomfort which he may be suffering are mitigated for the patient by the fact that he is regarded as 'lucky to be alive', a definition supported by all who surround him. He finds himself within a new pattern of living, structured for him by three groups of 'significant others' – the members of one group strangely changed in their relationships to him and two other groups previously unknown. His family and members of his social network, including representatives from his work situation, now appear only in short concentrated sessions and unfamiliar outdoor clothing. Whereas previously they demanded from him co-operation in many instrumental roles, now they are mainly limited to performing expressive roles in relation to him, while at the same time some of them will be taking on his previous instrumental roles at home and at work, thus altering previous definitions concerning his indispensability.

Men in this series did not lack visitors in hospital: in addition to wives, one third were visited by members of four different network categories (their own kin, wife's kin, children and non-kin); a further two out of every five had visitors from three of these categories as well as wives; and only two men received visits from no more than one category in addition to wives. If all members of their social networks had not already met, visiting hour in the hospital corridor appeared to provide occasion not only for meeting but also for interaction – 'Granny', said one woman, referring to her husband's mother, 'stands at the door and lets them through two at a time.' As we have already seen, some wives, having reason to fear lest anyone should 'say the wrong thing' or 'ask too many questions', tried to discourage excessive visiting, not always successfully.

Definitions made by family and network members, however, only impinge on patients for a very minor part of each day and, in the unfamiliar setting, are likely to carry relatively little authority. For definitions of the meaning of their physical symptoms patients are dependent on the staff, as they are for initial interpretations of the effect that the infarction may have on other aspects of their future lives. Here, it may not always be the most senior consultant who has the greatest impact; one woman described her husband as receiving most reassurance and detailed advice from a temporary ward orderly who had himself recovered from an infarction.

Staff are, however by no means the only new 'significant others' met in the ward. As patients recover they spend an increasing proportion of their time in observation of, or interaction with, fellow patients and this can affect the way that they come to see their own illness. Sometimes this may be in a positive way: more than one wife spoke of a husband becoming more determined to stop smoking after listening to heavy smokers 'groaning and coughing all night'. Sometimes, however, men compared their own treatment and progress with that of others and worried, in the absence of explanation, as to why some treatment prescribed for someone else was not given to them.

The social space created by hospitalisation and convalescence also provides unaccustomed free time for introspection and self-questioning. In this time there appeared to be a fairly widespread tendency to seek for a cause, acknowledged even by those who reported that they 'thought and thought and couldn't pin it on anything'. To a considerable extent such searching is fostered by the enquiries of 'significant others' who expect patients to be able to explain how and why their heart attack happened. Thus it is not enough for doctors to assume that patients have understood and accepted the explanations given to them unless they also feel capable of reproducing an explanation acceptable to their family and friends.

Although the search for causation was not a main focus for this study, we recognised that beliefs of patients and significant others about causal or contributory factors could hardly fail to impinge on the course of their post-infarction careers. Patients seemed to be attempting to 'make sense' out of the unexpected, to locate it in a biographical process — in effect, to put it into a 'career context' within definitions acceptable to prevalent ways of thinking. Their beliefs largely reflected common lay conceptions regarding causative factors, especially the idea of excess in work or in leisure activities as being stressful. The relative importance which they accorded to various factors associated with onset of illness are shown in Table 7.1. Very few men pointed to an immediately preceding activity. Only two described themselves as having been engaged in strenuous activity at the time, one cutting down a tree, one working with concrete; two others had finished strenuous activities — dancing and furniture moving respectively — shortly before becoming ill; half reported that they were going about routine activities and the remainder were sitting or resting at the onset of acute symptoms. The very normality of the immediately preceding state made the infarction all the more puzzling to them.

While two out of every five could point to no beliefs about associated factors, an equal number thought the illness was associated with their work. Very few named leisure activities although one in four mentioned other factors. Of those who did name some factor nearly one quarter named more than one. Only 8 per cent of the men and 11 per cent of their wives mentioned smoking as a cause or contributory factor : this despite the publicity already accorded at that time to the possible association between smoking and coronary heart disease (smoking habits of both spouses are discussed in Chapter 9).

Wives' views were, in general, similar to those of their husbands in the order in which they ranked different factors; however, they were much more positive, only a few having no ideas at all about causation. Work was indicted by seven out of every ten, leisure activities by one out of every five and other factors by two out of every five, the latter including heredity, overweight and personality.

The ability to point to a cause or contributory factor that had been temporary or was easily modifiable appeared to indicate a hopeful trajectory. Where patients could identify no possible factors or only factors which they considered difficult or impossible to alter then the possibilities for constructive adaptation seemed likely to be more limited.

Structuring of Services in Hospital and Community

Some studies, among them Dominian and Dobson,[1] have suggested that systems of intensive coronary care, involving sophisticated monitoring devices may cause or contribute to anxiety, fear and introspection, as well as fostering dependency. Only a few men in this series were taken to an Intensive Care Unit but among them we found no evidence to support this suggestion. This finding is in accordance with those of Cay and her colleagues[2] who, working with larger numbers in Edinburgh, found no evidence of adverse psychological effects, but who pointed to the need for caution in the interpretation of results from different coronary units. It seems that where staff are aware of these risks they can both reassure patients and start weaning them from the intensive care situation almost from the beginning so that undue dependence does not have a chance to develop.

In Dundee praise was almost uniformly high both for treatment in the Intensive Care Unit from those who went there and for treatment in the wards from the series as a whole. As one woman explained, her husband felt, when several hospital staff were all working to save him, 'If they are doing so much for me, I've got to help myself pull through' and others clearly had found reassurance in the quality of the care concentrated on them in the earliest stages of the post-infarction career.

The sense of gratitude to the staff, coupled with sheer joy at having survived — at having been 'one of the lucky ones' — helps to carry patients and their families over into the next phase of the post-infarction career when, after discharge, the long-term implications of the illness begin to loom larger and when optimism often begins to falter.

The stay by nearly one third of the men in the local convalescent hospital immediately following discharge from the acute ward did not appear to have any appreciable effect on attitudes or outcome, this form of treatment being largely determined by divergences in the policy of different units. One unit kept patients in the acute ward slightly longer and seldom used the convalescent hospital, while another unit kept patients a shorter time and sent most to the convalescent hospital for a week.

Despite occasional criticisms of inadequate appointment systems, in general the favourable attitudes developed by patients to treatment in hospital extended to cover both continued drug therapy and visits to outpatient clinics after discharge. At discharge, four out of every five were on treatment with drugs other than anticoagulants and one out of five were on anticoagulants, although there was some overlapping. Altogether, one third were on one drug only, over one in five were on two, one quarter on three, one in six on four and one man on five drugs. There was an association, as might be expected, between the number of drugs and the severity of the illness. Six months later, despite some minor changes, (a few men stopping drug therapy and a few starting) three out of every five who had been on treatment at discharge were still on treatment. Thus, in respect of drug treatment, there was a period of settling down and adjustment to reach a situation of reasonable stability by about six months. Most men appeared very conscientious in keeping to drugs prescribed for regular use and quickly learned how to adjust the use of those prescribed for specific contingencies, e.g. trinitrate for anginal pain, as well as sedatives and tranquillisers for 'when things get on top of me' or 'if I feel excited'. Where drug treatment, at least on a regular basis, was stopped at the time of return to work the two events were often linked in patients' minds as indications of recovery. Those who were on anticoagulant treatment made frequent and regular visits to hospital and, on these occasions, sometimes problems other than those directly associated with the control of their anticoagulant tablets were discussed informally (see Table 7.2).

Excluding anticoagulant control, the number of visits made to outpatient clinics ranged up to six. Nearly one quarter of the men were not considered to require outpatient visits, nearly half attended once or twice and the remainder between four and six times. The first appointment was usually made for about six weeks after discharge. Attendance at outpatient clinics did not appear to be related to the severity of the illness but rather to the patients' state at time of discharge and possibly to the policy of the consultant. Older patients also attended more frequently for follow-up. There were relatively few hospital readmissions within six months, only 9 per cent having one or more readmissions for further heart trouble and 6 per cent having admissions for other conditions. (see Table 7.3)

Much greater discontinuity and much greater variety in the patterns of care occurred in respect of contact with general practitioners. We have already seen that wives' expectations suggest that many men would be reluctant to approach their general practitioner. Their anxieties appeared justified and often did not seem to have been counterbalanced by active approaches from the doctors.

Approximately half of the patients did not receive home visits. Some men did not either expect one nor think that it was necessary; others, however, would have welcomed at least one home visit, preferably shortly after discharge since at this stage many felt very weak, tired and uncertain about what they should and could do. The experience of this series ranged from one man who received weekly home visits from his general practitioner to another who did not see his general practitioner at all. On discharge this patient telephoned to tell his doctor that he was perfectly well, arranging to telephone again if necessary. As he remained well and, being self-employed, required no certificates, he sought no further contact.

Altogether, approximately one man in every six reported receiving one home visit during the first six months, a slightly lower proportion reporting either two or three visits and a slightly higher proportion reporting more than three. Larger numbers of patients visited surgeries: excluding those made solely for the collection of repeat prescriptions, the number of surgery visits most frequently made was four, this being reported by over one quarter, while a similar proportion made fewer than four visits and nearly half between five and ten visits.

Contact with other services can only be described as minimal. Only seven men had seen a medical social worker while in hospital. One man had attended a resettlement clinic at the hospital following discharge and saw the Disablement Resettlement Officer from the Department of Employment on that occasion. Four men attended a rehabilitation or similar unit and six men were seen by the Regional Medical Officer within six months. A further three attended the Department of Employment (two seeing the Disablement Resettlement Officer) to seek a change of employment. There was virtually no use of other social agencies or voluntary organisations. This, despite evidence of considerable anxiety over modification and change in employment (see Chapter 8).

Hospital notes and copies of discharge letters sent to general practitioners contained, in most cases, fairly detailed summaries of patients' initial condition, progress, hospital treatment, condition at discharge and continuing treatment. They made, however, relatively little mention of advice in practical areas — diet being mentioned in only 6 per cent of the letters, smoking in 11 per cent and activity in 20 per cent.

This does not mean that such advice was not given. As can be seen from Table 7.4, patients remembered receiving considerably more advice than is indicated in the hospital notes. However, the lack of recorded notes means that there is difficulty either at the outpatient clinic (when a different doctor may see the patient), or at a subsequent readmission (perhaps to a different ward or hospital) in learning what advice has been given at earlier stages in the post-infarction career and, equally important, how the patient has responded to that advice. Similarly, there is little transmission of the stance taken by the hospital to the general practitioner, who has responsibility for maintaining care and giving continuing advice. In a condition when there is uncertainty about individual capability and the effect of behavioural changes much clearer recorded advice would appear to be desirable. This also applies to the recording at outpatients clinics, which usually take place about six weeks after discharge. Here, hospital notes recorded discussion on the following subjects — diet, 6 per cent, smoking 15 per cent, activity 56 per cent.

One of the four medical units routinely gave to post-infarction patients a leaflet setting out general guidelines to follow on discharge including advice on return to work, smoking, diet, resumption of sexual intercourse, exercise and car driving. It would be reasonable to suppose that in this unit it would not be deemed necessary to record detail on these these matters since the leaflet remained as a basis both for reference by the patient and for discussion between him and the general practitioner. However, another unit in the same hospital which did not issue a leaflet recorded very little more advice than the unit doing so. One patient who received the leaflet after readmission remarked that he wished he had been given it after his first infarction in another ward and his wife thought that the guidance it contained might have helped to prevent his second infarction.

Generally, men were given some indication, at an early stage of their illness, of the length of time they were likely to be off work thus being protected from the stresses of an indeterminate sentence and able to construct a timetable of recovery with a clear end point — return to work. Those who were not given this information (approximately one in four) would have preferred to have been told.

Most men agreed that they received some advice regarding activity, but often felt that this tended to be too general in character or, sometimes, rather contradictory, e.g. 'take plenty of exercise', 'don't get too tired', 'return to normal', 'gradually take up your former activities'. In a few instances, the advice was just not practicable, as illustrated by the general practitioner who advised a patient living half way up a very steep hill 'to walk on the level'. As he had been told not to drive and his wife did not drive, he could not even reach low ground. Similarly, advice to avoid cold winds appeared to make outdoor exercise less practicable for those whose post-infarction career began in winter.

The high percentage of men who received no advice on social and personal activities, as well as on diet, appears to reflect particular uncertainty among the medical profession on these areas. These are precisely the areas most affected by social class and other cultural differences and it may be that doctors avoid them because they lack knowledge of different customs and attitudes or alternatively they may fail to communicate clearly with patients.

Patient-Doctor Transactions

We have already suggested that feelings of relief at survival and appreciation of hospital care at the acute stage tend to carry patients and their families over into the next stage. Towards the end of the hospital stay the men themselves were making optimistic definitions of the situation and visualising fewer problems than did their wives. Indeed half were quite emphatic that there would be no problems whatsoever about return to work and very few indeed described themselves as very worried about their future or their employment.

Six months later however, there was evidence of considerable dissatisfaction. For many the optimistic definitions made at discharge no longer seemed to apply and such contact as they maintained with outpatient clinics and general practitioners was failing to resolve the uncertainties and confusion felt by these men and their wives. In particular, there were complaints about lack of information and difficulties in communicating with doctors, especially over matters which were important to patients but which they felt were considered to be trivial by doctors. The limitations of a poor relationship were illustrated by one man who, in the course of a research interview six months after discharge, enquired whether he would be well enough to go abroad for his holiday in two months' time. When (in accordance with our policy), it was suggested that he should discuss this with his own doctor, he said 'I couldn't possibly ask him that — you don't know my doctor!'

From the patient's perspective, lack of consistent information in these areas leads to uncertainty and anxiety and leaves him exposed to negative influences emanating both from folklore and earlier professional attitudes out of phase with current medical thought. In connection with such a common disease, particularly in a series such as this where just over three out of every four patients had some family history of heart trouble, tales of other sufferers and usually those with a poor outcome, are common. The tales are likely to refer predominantly to past decades when a more cautious and negative approach was adopted by doctors and thus comments like 'he was never the same again' reflect fairly accurately the end result of previous care régimes.

Monteiro[3] has examined expectations among the general population in Rhode Island concerning the behaviour of post-infarction patients and has shown how this is modified by age and personal experience of heart disease. While the general lay view was favourable towards activity for the post-infarction patient, rejecting the idea that he should be restricted to leading a passive life, those · with experience of heart disease themselves or who knew someone who had experienced it were also those who inclined towards belief in the need for restriction of activity. Younger people and those of a higher educational level and a higher income level were, however, found to be

more favourable towards activity. Monteiro's findings illustrate the
way in which innovation in medical care is differentially accepted
according to an individual's existing framework of knowledge.

It is sometimes suggested that the absence of a 'family doctor'
responsible for treating both spouses may be important in recovery
from serious illness. In this series, seven in every ten couples attended
the same general practitioner while nearly half of the remainder
normally attended doctors within the same practice. Non-manual
families and incomers more often attended the same doctor than did
manual families and sedentes; for some of the latter the question of
changing from the practice attended during childhood had never arisen.
There was no direct evidence that the absence of a family doctor or a
family practice was, in itself, important in determining attitudes or
outcome. Nevertheless, it did add one more barrier to ease of
communication and consistency of advice for a minority of families,
and, relatively more often, for those already disadvantaged in
other respects.

In general, however, the actual structuring of services appeared of
less importance than the quality of communication between doctor and
patient and doctor and family. A small minority, having adequate
'room to manoeuvre' in social and occupational roles and enjoying
support from social networks whose definitions were congruent with
professional definitions needed little help in accepting new 'recipes
for action' and incorporating them into new and satisfactory self-
concepts. The majority however, found this a disturbing and
discouraging process, many abandoning some or all attempts at
adaptation. Those who most needed help were often the most
reluctant to seek it and appeared least able to articulate doubts and
uncertainties. Specific recipes for action often contributed to a
sense of loss and discontinuity which accorded ill with the more
general advice to 'get back to normal'.

Notes

1. Dominian, J. and Dobson, M. (1969). Study of Patients' Psychological
   Attitudes to a Coronary Care Unit. *British Medical Journal* 4, 795-8.
2. Cay, E.L., Vetter, N., Philip, A.E. and Dugard, P. (1972). Psychological
   Reactions to a Coronary Care Unit. *Journal of Psychosomatic Research*
   16, 437-47.
3. Monteiro, A. (1973). After Heart Attack: Behavioral Expectations for the
   Cardiac. *Social Science and Medicine* 7, 555-65.

Return to work is usually taken as the simplest objective criterion of recovery. Overall, 78 per cent of the men in this series achieved this at six months, a figure very similar to those in studies of comparable populations. Such apparently good results may, however, mask considerable difficulties and problems facing those who return. It is also important to consider why delay in returning and failure to return occur and what they mean to the individual.

Garrity,[1] in his study of vocational adjustment after first myocardial infarction, has reviewed the American literature on determinants of return to work. His findings, emphasising the importance both of the patient's health perception and the pressures of significant others, lead him to support the need for rehabilitation counselling for cardiac patients.

Roth,[2] studying tuberculosis patients, demonstrated the process of negotiation in recovery, particularly in respect of the timetabling of events. Return to work after any serious illness may involve considerable negotiation and decision-making to which the patient himself, his doctor and family members may all contribute, as well as employers, fellow employees and friends. Current emphasis by the medical profession on speedy return to work (this itself often being regarded as therapeutic) may be counterbalanced by norms in the community operating in the direction of caution. There are also work situations where gradual return is not possible or where full fitness is required, for instance, heavy manual work, solitary occupations and those which carry responsibility for others.

When return is achieved, continuing redefinition of the situation may occur for a considerable time. Further recovery may be less than was hoped, the period providing for initial work modifications may not prove long enough and unexpected difficulties may arise. Many individuals in the occupational setting — managers, foremen, union representatives, team mates, industrial medical advisers and others — may participate in the changing situation, each contributing different definitions influenced by their own interests or by the interests of those whom they represent.

Pre-Infarction Employment Background

For this series of men, the local economic situation at the time of
infarction was not conducive to reassurance. The city, with a
population of approximately 180,000, is still very dependent on the
jute industry and, to a lesser extent, on heavy engineering despite the
advent of light engineering industries and electronic developments,
which have provided greater diversity since the Second World War.
It has always been highly vulnerable to economic difficulties and the
beginning of the study in 1970 coincided with a period of economic
recession which was particularly evident in the Dundee area. High
unemployment meant that the threat of redundancy was very real for
many people, as is seen in the study. Later the economic situation
gradually improved, with the development of North Sea Oil
contributing to this.

As indicated in Chapter 4, only four men in this series were
unemployed at the time of infarction and other one was not
working because of illness. Overall, more than half had experienced a
stable occupational record over the previous five years and fewer than
one in ten had made frequent changes. Never the less, uncertainties
and dissatisfaction lay beneath the surface for many. It became clear
during interviews that about one in every five had become aware of the
threat of redundancy at varying stages in the months preceding
infarction. Some had received notice, others were expecting it. Most
had not thought to mention this in hospital and they had not been
asked about it by those treating them. In addition, slightly more than
half of all men were dissatisfied with some aspect of their employment
at that time, 14 per cent claiming that they had not been physically
able to manage their work and an equal number admitting to some
difficulties in managing, while 17 per cent described themselves as
not completely content with their work and another 6 per cent
experienced some difficulties with fellow workers. The remainder
felt quite confident in hospital that there would be no difficulties over
return to work. (Table 8.1)

Variables Related to Return

Table 8.2 in the Appendix shows some details of occupational
outcome at six months in relation to severity of infarction, social
class and age. It will be seen that, in respect of return to former
employment, differential outcome varies more between different
social classes and ages than between grades of severity, with men in
Social Classes I and II and intermediate age groups being much more

likely to return to their former employment and men in Classes IV and V and youngest age groups much less likely.

Attitudes to work before infarction did not seem to make much difference, all those previously unhappy at work having returned and most of those who had previously been experiencing difficulties; however, the proportion who returned among those who anticipated post-infarction difficulties while in hospital was somewhat lower — just under two out of every three.

Medical Advice on Return to Work

Advice was classified as specific when men were told that they were definitely able, or unable, to return to their former employment; and as general when it was limited to restrictions such as 'take it easy', 'don't get too tired', or 'don't do heavy lifting'. Table 8.3 shows that nearly half received no appreciable advice and considered that they had no discussion with a doctor on their work, apart from the actual timing of their return which generally required certification. Altogether, approximately one in every six was advised on a permanent change of work or working conditions, nearly one quarter were advised to have a temporary change and one in ten was told to have a trial to see if the work could be managed. Direct approaches by doctors to employers on a patient's behalf were made in two instances only.

Men were asked whether they had discussed their illness in relation to their work with anyone in their previous, or new, employment. Overall, three out of every five had discussed this with some non-medical person in a position of responsibility. Despite the fact that nearly one third of the men were employed in establishments having a regular occupational health service, only three individuals were seen by any medical personnel at their place of employment before starting work, these three all being seen both by an occupational health service doctor and a nurse, an arrangement which could, surely, be more widely used.

Timing, Work Modifications and Difficulties

Of the 62 men who were working at six months, nearly one half (45 per cent) had started by three months. This is in accordance with the findings of other studies, in particular Sharland[3] who recorded 55 per cent as returning to work at three months and 82 per cent at six months; Groden[4], recording 44 per cent at three and 82 per cent at six months; and Wincott and Caird[5] recording 58 per cent at

three months and 83 per cent at six months. The latter went on to
record 88 per cent at twelve months (however, as we see in Chapter
10, the proportion of men working at twelve months in this series had
fallen to 74 per cent, a few men not working at six months having
returned but others working at that time being ill at twelve months).

Even by six months, there were indications of changes having taken
place both in health perception and in employment status between
three and six months which suggest that optimism associated with
early return may not always be sustained without continuing
support from medical services and within the work situation. (Table 8.4)

Work was modified, at least temporarily, for two out of every
three returned workers. At six months nearly one half were still
working reduced hours while the remainder had reverted to normal
hours (apart from three men who were working longer hours than
before). Reduction in hours was associated with the physical nature
of previous work, nearly two out of every three heavy workers reducing
their hours while only one quarter of light workers did so. There was
also some indication that reduction was associated with severity of
infarct, previous general illness and the man's belief that work had
been a causal factor in onset.

Just under one third claimed to have felt no difficulty in starting
work and, among these, one in every eight felt that they could have
started earlier if they had been encouraged to do so. Of the
remainder, half had only transient difficulty as after any illness while
the other half experienced considerable difficulties initially. (Table 8.5)

By six months, 5 per cent were on sickness benefit and unable to
work: 12 per cent continued working despite definite and serious
difficulties; 13 per cent experienced less serious difficulties and felt
that they could manage their work reasonably well; and another
9 per cent thought that the work that they were doing was not really
in accordance with the medical advice which they had received. There
was a significant association between having post-infarction difficulties
at work and having post-infarction angina. Some indication of an
association between having difficulties and having suffered previous
symptoms of general illness (not heart disease) appeared to exist;
men whose work was classified as moderate appeared more often to
experience difficulties than did those in heavy or light work. No
association was found between difficulties and severity of
infarct, age or the belief that work was a causal factor in onset.

Post-infarction Occupational Change

Of the five men who changed work as a result of the illness all
but one appeared to benefit from the change. A cattleman, who had
been doing long hours and undertaking additional casual work, was
advised by the hospital doctor to look for an alternative occupation and
was referred to the Disablement Resettlement Officer who could offer
him nothing. However, he found work for himself as an industrial spray
painter. This necessitated giving up his tied house but he managed to
obtain a council house, probably partly because his wife and one of his
young children also had health problems. He was quite satisfied with
his new work and with the move.

A skilled tradesman who was unemployed at the time of
infarction had previously experienced a chequered work record
associated with chronic alcoholism. After recovery from infarction he
signed on at the Department of Employment but was not referred to
the Disablement Resettlement Officer and was offered no work. Then,
through a friend, he applied for work in his original trade in a large
firm. In applying he admitted to being an alcoholic (because, as he
said, this was known in the trade) but made no mention of his heart
trouble, seemingly feeling that any stigma associated with his long-
standing disability would be less discouraging to employers than that
associated with heart disease — or perhaps that admitting to one
disability was sufficient especially since he could use it to explain his
stay in hospital. His application was successful and he was pleased
with the new job. His wife, when she was seen later reported that his
alcoholism worried her so much that his heart condition seemed of less
importance.

A carpenter in a contracting firm was paid off while ill but asserted
that this did not worry him since this type of work is never secure and
he had been accustomed to moving frequently from firm to firm.
He readily found himself work in another firm, having made no
contact with the Department of Employment, and expressed himself
as very content with the change. However as we see in Chapter 10, he
had a second heart attack before twelve months and, although he was
able to return to work with his new firm, his wife felt that his life
was endangered by his resistance to seeking medical help lest he be
put off work again.

Although no man in this series who required change of employment
had in fact been placed in work at six months by the Department of
Employment, one man, who was previously a salesman, was
undergoing government-sponsored training as a clerk. This appeared

to be the only example of successful intervention by non-medical services, and as we see later his wife thought that this had brought to light talents which he had previously denied possessing.

A less happy story came from a man who had been for many years in stable employment. Latterly, his work as foreman had exposed him to considerable stress and, for some time before infarction, he had been consulting his general practitioner from whom he had understood that it would be advisable to change to a less demanding occupation. Having sought and been offered work in a different trade, he had just given up his old job but had not yet begun his new one when he fell ill. During his time in hospital he was told that the new job could not be kept for him and he was thus unemployed at time of discharge. He had been referred by the ward sister to the medical social worker, who arranged a resettlement clinic at the hospital and thus he had come into contact with the Disablement Resettlement Officer. However, the only suggestion that the latter was able to offer was assessment in an industrial rehabilitation unit. He rejected this and applied for approximately twenty jobs before getting one as a van salesman which he found tiring. At six months he was considering retraining but was still working as a van salesman at twelve months; his wife felt that he had received no help and said that 'there had been no rehabilitation'.

Most of the fifteen men who had expected to be made redundant were, in fact working at three months, ten of them with their former employer and two in another firm. Two of those who had returned to their former employer were subsequently made redundant and had not found other work at six months. Others believed that it was partly because of their illness that threatened redundancy had not been effected.

Of the two men who retired, a Fire Service Officer aged 56, had suffered his infarction just a few weeks before he was due to retire. He had been planning to take part-time work after retirement and found a suitable opportunity between six and twelve months. A manager, who worked in a very demanding industry, had not made up his mind what to do when, shortly after his discharge from hospital, he received fairly severe injuries in a road accident for which he was in no way responsible. He then retired early, attributing this mainly to the disability resulting from the accident. (His wife, however had expressed her hope that he would retire after the infarction.) Another man, a shopkeeper, lost his business by compulsory purchase while ill. At six months he felt quite well, helped his working wife with their young family and was quite content. (At twelve months, however, under pressure from the Department of Health and Social Security, he was about to start work in sheltered conditions.)

Three of the men who had not returned to work by six months had either been unemployed or declared redundant before infarction and one had been off work for some time with pre-existing illness (these four were all normally in semi- or unskilled occupations). Several more had work being kept open for them but were not well enough to return at six months. The two bus drivers in this series had very divergent experiences. One was told that he could not return to his former work and, despite efforts to obtain alternative employment, was still on sickness benefit at six and twelve months; like the shopkeeper who lost his business he had a young family and helped his working wife. In contrast, another bus driver, who suffered what was described in the medical notes as an 'appalling' infarct and who was very ill in hospital, had returned to regular bus driving (in a different company) with no difficulty.

Return to Work as a Transition

The experience of this series suggests that the relatively high rates of return should not cause complacency. Some of the minority who did not return might have done so if they had received more positive intervention early in the post-infarction career aimed at preventing a drift into unemployability. Others for whom return seemed less feasible could still have benefited from sheltered employment, occupational therapy or involvement with voluntary organisations. For men whose previous self-image has often been strongly dependent on their work-role, the change to being even temporarily idle can be very traumatic, particularly in manual occupations where the importance of physical strength and the male role as breadwinner are stressed.

Our findings are in accordance with those of Groden and Cheyne[6] who reported that only a tiny minority of unemployed cardiacs attending an assessment clinic were workshy. They found that more than half were unemployed because of a combination of psychological and environmental factors and minor physical symptoms or as a result of the attitudes and anxieties of immediate family, family doctor or employer.

For the majority who do return to work, the issue is not a simple one. The very fact of returning is, in general, a change of positive, reassuring significance but the timing of return requires more detailed consideration as does the need for sustained support providing continuity from hospital discharge and directed towards making return as early and as anxiety-free as possible. In this series it was clear that some men were very inadequately prepared for return, which came as a sudden shock with considerable initial difficulties. In the early days of return some contemplated premature retirement.

There were indications that doctors tend to think of a man's limitations in a purely physiological and functional way rather than trying to visualise the implications which they may have on his social roles and particularly his work role. Doctors also often lack knowledge of industrial work and may play for safety by advising 'light work' without enquiring more carefully into what is involved in the patient's usual work. Perhaps some are hesitant to reveal their ignorance of industrial processes but they would usually find that to ask the patient about his work in detail (and sometimes about alternatives as he sees them) can initiate a very constructive dialogue which should increase the doctor's awareness of likely contingencies while at the same time improving his relationship with the patient and bringing to the surface anxieties often suppressed.

The characteristics of a man's work are not always self-evident from its title. For instance, the work of a postman is generally considered to provide healthy exercise and, as a well-known educational film on heart disease emphasises, postmen as a group have low rates of myocardial infarction. However, a postman in this series alternated two weeks of van delivery with one of foot delivery; since he covered a small town built on unusually steep hills, the contrast between the exercise he took in different weeks was extreme. In his case, temperament also appeared to operate to his disadvantage, his wife describing him as 'always hashing on as if there wasna another day — if he were to be a minute late that widna do'. She added that the compulsion was in his nature rather than the nature of the work. Other men appeared equally time-driven or conscientious beyond the seeming demands of their work and, for these, it would seem that adjustment of work conditions would need to be accompanied by skillful counselling.

Goble and his colleagues[7] have reported from Australia that to describe a patient as fit for light work, restricted duties or part-time work only is often 'a passport to unemployment'. This, they explain, throws the responsibility on

the employer, the personnel officer or the foreman. He cannot
accept this responsibility although he usually does his best. It is the
doctor's responsibility to find out the exact nature of the job and
to decide whether the patient can do it — and if not, what
modifications are required. Usually the patient will be able to give
the answer himself, but all too often he is not asked.

It would seem valuable to provide for the possibility, where patients
agree, of discussion between doctor and employer; this would give the
employer the appropriate information if conditions need to be varied
and would at the same time reassure him about safety in relation to
any particular job. This contact could equally well be made by a
hospital doctor, a general practitioner or a rehabilitation officer who
knows the patient. Brewerton[8] gives a useful account of what can be
achieved by a Hospital Rehabilitation Officer in this context. These
contacts also provide a way of educating employers and others in a
positive approach to rehabilitation and can help them explain it to
others in the work team. Such discussion can be most easily achieved
where there is an occupational health service; this service can also
provide the benefit of immediate help and support through the early
period of return to work for the patient and the firm.

Doctors may need to carry particular responsibilities in relation to
the self-employed man because, in these circumstances there is no one
other than himself (and possibly partners, sometimes including
family members) to define the situation and to help work out
alterations. On the face of it, the lot of the self-employed man often
appears to offer an ideal situation for gradual recovery. In this series
this appeared to be true for men with suitable professions or
prosperous businesses who had plenty of 'room for manoeuvre'; men
in marginally viable businesses were, however, exposed to considerable
strains and so were their wives.

Overall, opportunities for positive role rearrangement in the work
situation appeared to be fewer than might have been expected from
the serious nature of the illness as well as from the sense of shock and
the good intentions present at the time of hospitalisation. What did
seem to dominate the definitions of both men and their wives was a
sense of role loss or diminution, generally with little sense of positive
gain to counterbalance this.

Men in flexible non-manual occupations appeared to experience
this sense of role loss or diminution less often. More of them could
arrange their work setting to suit themselves; consequently, where

role change was needed, by initiating it themselves they were more able to perceive adaptation in positive terms. This was well exemplified by a senior professional man who 'phased hinself down to equal terms with his junior partner' as part of a long-term plan towards retirement. His wife explained that he was glad to be able to give to his partner an easier introduction to seniority than he himself had experienced years before when the sudden death of *his* senior partner had precipitated him into sudden overwhelming responsibility and the habit of long-term overwork. This man also had very satisfying spare-time commitments in the community which would sustain his self-esteem.

No doubt having 'room to manoeuvre' was important to employers also. One woman spoke of her husband's employers as rearranging the work 'because there have been too many heart attacks and other illnesses'; but another woman said that, although there had once been a few lighter jobs available in the firm where her husband was employed in a managerial capacity, they were now all occupied by other employees with disabilities.

Occasionally, there was evidence of unexpected role gain, modification of the social construction of reality appearing to play a part in this process. A salesman had changed to clerical work and was working towards a professional qualification through evening classes. His wife said

> In a funny sort of way, it's turned out a good thing because it's brought to light talents he had not known existed and he has a chance now to make something quite good of his life. Otherwise he'd have been trudging on as usual. I had suggested years ago he should leave saleswork and go to night school but he always said he wasn't brainy and hadn't confidence. Now he says he was pushed into it and is glad because he would never had done it otherwise.

She expressed reservations, however, about his continued heavy smoking and diet difficulties which suggested some discontinuity between the positive qualities of adaptability which he had displayed in his occupational career and negative characteristics which she saw as still hindering his health career. (In fact, as is shown in Chapter 14, this man had a second infarction later, after which he made the other adjustments required.)

Positive success in occupational adaptation was however very much a minority pattern and, even for men with favourable outcomes, many wives still expressed reservations a year later. Some were conscious of changed economic conditions threatening their husbands and the interaction of such threats with his health and changed medical record, sometimes indicating that they themselves were in the process of reordering experience. The wife of a professional man in a small business said that her husband had received notice of redundancy eleven months after infarction. He had not said much but she thought 'he looked worse for two to three days than at any time during his illness. For a week I had to bolster his ego along; then, we went away for a weeks' camping holiday and he got things back into proper perspective.' She added

> Now I'm beginning to see his work in a new light. Before, there was nothing you could put your finger on but I had a feeling for a time that he wasn't getting anywhere, that he was frustrated. There was promise in the firm but I didn't see it being fulfilled — there was nothing definite but little things made me wonder. When he said he was to go I said 'Are you really sorry?' and he said 'No'. Somehow it wasn't a shock to me. I seem to have foreseen it all. He was not working to his potential. It's a funny thing but our son said the same when he heard he was to go.

This woman had not mentioned any doubts at first interview.

A business man's wife said that her husband's firm had been taken over and although 'he wouldn't have worried about the takeover before his illness', he did now for 'where would he get a job with his age and medical record of a heart attack?' The takeover had only been a possibility before his illness but now 'everyone has seen the light at the end of the tunnel and it's not a very nice light — you can always adapt, but it's the fear of the unknown that gives you a nasty feeling in the pit of your stomach'. She added that it was for this reason, rather than as any direct effect of the illness itself, that they had moved house and had cut down on social activities and that she herself was trying to get a job. Implicitly, she was defining her husband's career as the major current worry but acknowledging that his prospects had meanwhile been affected by the illness and its effect of labelling him with an adverse medical record. (At first interview she had indicated a degree of doubt about the work setting, saying 'It's hard to know how the firm will react, especially with business the way it is.')

Thus work settings and work roles, already somewhat problematic for at least half the men in this series before infarction, now appeared to contain overt or underlying threats for many. This made the satisfactions afforded by leisure roles all the more important and we look at these in the next chapter.

Notes

1. Garrity, T.F. (1973). Vocational Adjustment after First Myocardial Infarction; Comparative Assessment of Several Variables Suggested in the Literature. *Social Science and Medicine* 7, 705-17.
2. Roth, J.A. (1963). *Timetables*, Indianapolis, Bobbs-Merrill.
3. Sharland, D.E. (1964). Ability of Men to Return to Work After Cardiac Infarction. *British Medical Journal* 2, 718-20.
4. Groden, B.M. (1967). Return to Work After Myocardial Infarction. *Scottish Medical Journal* 12, 297-301.
5. Wincott, E.A. and Caird, F.I. (1966). Return to Work after Myocardial Infarction. *British Medical Journal* 2, 1302-4.
6. Groden, B.M. and Cheyne, A.I. (1972). Rehabilitation After Cardiac Illness. *British Medical Journal* 2, 700-703.
7. Goble, A.J., Adey, G.M. and Bullen, J.F. (1963). Rehabilitation of the Cardiac Patient. *The Medical Journal of Australia* 2, 975-82.
8. Brewerton, D.A. and Daniel, J.W. (1969). Return to Work: Experiences of a Hospital Rehabilitation Officer. *British Medical Journal* 2, 240-42.

9 TRANSITION AND ADAPTATION: LOSS AND GAIN IN ROLES AND VALUES

We have seen in the previous chapter that four out of every five men had resumed work roles by six months after infarction. Change in other domains of living is less easy to assess but at six months there was considerable evidence of loss of role in social and physical activities and decrease in self-esteem and confidence, with only a small minority finding compensatory roles and new sources of self-esteem, and this was confirmed by interviews with wives at one year. Goffman[1] has described involuntary loss of role in a number of social situations and the resulting changes in the conception which the loser has of himself and the conception that others have of him. Although lack of rigid integration of a person's social roles may allow him to seek comfort in one role from injuries incurred in others, in some cases 'the shattering experience in one area of social life may spread out to all the sectors of his activity. He may define away the barriers between his several social roles and become a source of difficulty in all of them.' There were indications that, for many men in this series, the changed perception which they had of their health and consequently of themselves, amounted to just this kind of shattering experience spreading out into all sectors of activity.

Garrity[2] has stated that

the importance of clinical health status, especially severity of the attack, as a determinant of return to work and amount of work involvement may have been over-estimated. More important, at least in relation to return to work, may be the way in which the patient *sees* his health. This seems quite reasonable since clinical health status must be translated into the patient's understanding before it can be used as a factor in personal decision-making. The patient's perception of his health may be further shaped by personal biases and experiences, the physician's communications and other factors. This amalgamation called 'patient health perception' appears to be more powerful in determining return to work than any of its medical, social or psychological components.

We would agree that patient health perception is important in respect of return to work but this should not be taken to mean that all, or even the majority of, patients who return to work perceive their health in a favourable way, and, perhaps just as important, unfavourable patient health perception appears to be closely bound up with loss of role and quality of life in other spheres as well as work.

Health Perception

In this series only one in every four men described themselves as free of symptoms at three months while just over half reported angina and two out of every five mentioned other symptoms (some mentioned both angina and other symptoms, see Table 9.1). At six months the proportions were virtually unchanged, this being in fact the area in which least change between three and six months was reported. Of the patients who reported angina the proportion who were at work (48 per cent) was very little lower than it was among those not having angina (51 per cent). Many described vague complaints — 'a bit of an ache', 'a bit of tightness' or 'pain on exertion or if excited'. Whenever they experienced any symptom they tended to wonder if it was related to their heart condition even if this seemed unlikely, and, in general, they were more conscious of the state of their health.

There was frequently evidence of failure to report symptoms to doctors and of understatement of such symptoms when they were mentioned. This may well encourage the medical profession in the erroneous belief that all is well. Such denial or playing down of symptoms may be present even before discharge. One patient mentioned the man in the next bed to him who had been admitted with myocardial infarction on the same day and who continually complained to him of pain and other symptoms but on no occasion reported them to the staff. Both men were discharged on the same day. Our evidence is in agreement with that of Wishnie and his colleagues[3] who in 1971 described 'the tendency of the post-coronary patient to minimize symptoms and deny emotional troubles during follow-up visits with his physician' and who commented that this had not, to their knowledge been reported before.

If any particular activity produces pain or a sense of tightness many patients are discouraged from trying it again; alternatively, they may do so only after a prolonged period during which fitness has further declined or they may be in such a state of apprehension and tension as itself will foster symptoms. It is at such times that lay beliefs about the fragility of the heart and the potential harmfulness of activity are likely to rush in, pushing aside memories of medical advice which seems not applicable or not practical to that individual in that specific contingency.

The lay definition of cardiac illness has been described by Monteiro[4] as protecting the patient against the resumption of his normal role responsibilities rather than encouraging him to leave the sick role. Experience in this series suggests that lay definitions are likely to impinge all the more sharply because, unlike generalised medical advice, they are inevitably concerned with the immediate and the specific — the first decision for instance, as to whether to lift a piece of furniture or to go out in the first cold wind. Positive decisions may be seen as actions which carry risk of immediate penalties (pain, another attack, death) and which offer no immediate rewards. The alternative negative decisions (procrastination or abandonment) may be seen as involving no risks, losing no rewards and offering the compensation of having 'played for safety' or 'erring on the safe side'. Although some men and their families coped with these natural hesitations without undue difficulty, many others would have liked more detailed anticipation of specific contingencies and the opportunity to have medical advice reassessed or reinforced when unforeseen problems occurred. In particular they would have liked more guidance on resumption of sexual intercourse, car driving, long-distance travel, participation in sports and lifting heavy objects.

Physical and Social Activities

At six months after infarction, two out of every five reported that they were less physically active and had reduced participation in sports (Table 9.2). This appeared to be associated with older age groups, a mild infarction, continuing attendance at outpatient clinics and continuing drug treatment including anticoagulants. In particular, strenuous activities such as cycling, tennis, team sports and dancing had been reduced. Many men gave up decorating, household repairs or strenuous work in the garden, such activities generally being taken over by other family members. In a few instances the purchase of a powered lawn mower or a move to a house without a garden was an alternative solution.

Only a few men (about one in seven) reported increased physical activities. Generally this meant walking and golf, possibly reflecting medical opinions as to what constitutes suitable exercise. One manual worker taking to golf was joined by his son and son-in-law. Wives often

accompanied their husbands on walks at first but tended not to
continue. Favourable environment and weather had made it easier and
more pleasant for some men to begin and maintain daily walks. Car
owning and women's ability to drive had sometimes enabled others
to reach pleasant and varied surroundings. One couple achieved this at
an early stage despite very strong winter winds, the wife driving in the
direction of the wind so that her husband could walk home with the
wind behind him.

The remainder (approximately two out of every five) claimed to be
about as active as before infarction. Most of these admitted that, in
fact, they had been accustomed to taking hardly any exercise
and had reverted to this pattern, watching television being their only
pastime apart from occasional visits to pubs or relatives. A small
minority (approximately one in every six) had been active before
infarction, both mentally and physically. Some of these had found
that they needed to accept some reduction in activity or specific
strenuous activities, but this was often seen as temporary and they
looked forward to possible resumption at a later date, meanwhile
substituting compensatory activities (generally walking) to the fullest
extent possible.

Participation in social activity had also decreased for more than
half the men at three months and for over one third this still held
at six months. Decrease appeared to be associated with severity of
infarct, older age group, previous symptoms of heart disease,
especially angina, and continuing hospital care at outpatient clinics
as well as with the belief that leisure activities were involved in
causation. Some men had cut peripheral or optional activities such as
voluntary work and, sometimes, there was a tendency to limit the
total sphere of activities which, when taken in connection with
decrease in physical activity, seemed to result in a very narrow
pattern of living with little left except the work role. Another third
explained that they had previously taken very little part in social
activities and so this had been minimally affected by infarction.
In some instances wives described men as having reduced earlier
social activities long before infarction either because of specific
health problems or because of tiredness or lack of energy.

Problems and Difficulties

Six months after infarction over one third reported that the illness
had resulted in personal and/or social problems and one in five that
it had caused financial difficulties. Nearly one in three expressed

fears, either about the recurrence of a heart attack or about ability to cope in the future, and over half said that they had found it difficult to adapt. Some, however, who did not admit to fears added comments at various stages in interviews which suggested underlying fears which they resisted bringing to the surface. Where there was an obvious clear-cut problem such as inability to return to work, men often appeared to find it easier to admit their worries.

Feelings of uncertainty, fear and frustration appeared closely linked together. One man described himself as feeling 'alone in my uncertainty'. Others spoke of being 'frightened to do anything' or 'scared to do anything active'. For some this appeared to have led to an identity crisis in which they felt that they no longer knew what kind of person they were and doubted their future. Several expressed a lack of confidence in themselves or in their ability to cope with specific contingencies in work or leisure — responsibility, decision-making, concentration, mixing in company. One, who was still off work, said 'I am worried that I am on the scrap heap.' Another, who had returned, said that 'the thought of having had a heart attack is always with you but I don't tell anyone — I don't want to think about it'. Sometimes fear was specifically related to the frightening experience of the heart attack itself — 'I couldn't go through that again.' Virtually all the men knew someone who had experienced more than one attack and virtually all also knew someone who had died of a further attack.

Many had previously been very independent and hated the frustration and humiliation of being told by family members or workmates: 'don't do that — let me do it'. Sometimes, if alone, they would find themselves reverting to lifting a heavy weight or 'going hard at' some strenuous task and then, suddenly remembering, they would experience fear. It seemed that the advice 'you will be all right if you take it easy' was taken as implying 'you will kill yourself if you go hard at anything'.

Previous orientations and patterns of living affected the way in which different men coped with contingencies in the post-infarction career. For a small minority, the infarction provided occasion for a careful assessment of their way of life, after which they made some planned adjustments and were well satisfied; sometimes they admitted that they were more appreciative of life than ever before, while a few expressed surprise that they had been able to adapt and to find the results acceptable. These were men who had been generally active, both mentally and physically, before infarction and who

appeared to have 'room to manoeuvre' both in work and social roles.
Any adverse circumstances which were recognised as possibly
contributing to the infarction were not seen as immutable.

For another small number of men the impact of infarction
appeared to be lessened by the fact that previous disability or chronic
illness had already lowered expectations and provided practice in the
acceptance of limitations. A man who had previously had an arm
amputated said 'I did not get any help — I did not need any.'
Previous styles of adaptation were, however, not necessarily suited
to their new condition.

Another relatively small group of men who often described
themselves as not being 'the worrying kind' tended to go on after
infarction much as before — 'I take things much as they come' —
or to make only minor, generally decremental, changes — 'You've got
to accept that things are different and you have to take things
easily.' Such men were often among those who resisted advice on
exercise and smoking.

Much more common, however, were men who worried about the
effects of infarction without seeming to have the necessary 'room
for manoeuvre', either in psychological or social terms, to enable
constructive adaptations to be made. Such men often appeared to
have been extremely conscientious even obsessional, in regard to
work and social obligations before infarction. Sometimes there was
evidence of the crisis of hospitalisation, together with unexpected
serious illness, reactivating former feelings of anxiety, depression or
other personality problems.

Change in Smoking Habits

Smoking habits appeared very important, both as an indication of
dependence before infarction and resistance to, or acceptance of,
change after infarction. In this series over 84 per cent were smokers
at the time of infarction (Table 9.3). The Report of the Royal
College of Physicians in 1971[5] gives the percentage of males in
Britain who smoke as ranging from just under 60 to just over
70 per cent, depending on age. The higher percentage found in this
study would be expected in a disease which is associated with smoking.

Russell[6] has drawn attention to the nature and severity of
cigarette dependence. 'Cigarette smoking is probably the most
addictive and dependence producing form of object-specific
self-administered gratification known to men.'

Surveys have shown that three out of four current smokers either wish to or have tried to stop smoking yet only 15 per cent succeed in stopping smoking permanently before the age of 60.[7] Thus most people smoke not because they wish to but because they cannot easily stop. Only 2 per cent of smokers are able to limit themselves to intermittent or occasional smoking and the majority are regular dependent smokers who seldom go more than an hour or two without smoking.

Some knowledge of the risks of smoking is now widespread in Britain, largely as a result of the warning on cigarette packets introduced in 1971, combined with the ban on cigarette advertising on television which has been in force since 1965. The two reports by the Royal College of Physicians[8] received wide publicity. All patients in this series seemed aware that smoking is 'bad for your health' but by no means all understood what the effects were.

In common with a number of cities, anti-smoking clinics run by Local Health Authority Services have existed in Dundee since 1964. In the early years only just over one tenth of the population attending these clinics still abstained from smoking at six months but, in more recent clinics, the success rate at six months has risen to one third.[9]

Graham and Gibson[10] have examined some of the factors involved in cessation of smoking. Two of their hypotheses which were substantiated were that those who give up smoking are more likely to have been hospitalised recently and to have more accurate information concerning scientific findings on the harmful effects of smoking.

It might be thought that the incentive to stop and to remain a non-smoker would be greater after an illness such as myocardial infarction where a direct association with smoking can be shown, especially since health is generally cited as the main reason for wanting to stop and since hospitalisation often entails at least temporary cessation. Certainly, it would appear to provide an opportunity for professionals to intervene positively and to follow up results both in patients and family members.

A study in Edinburgh has shown the value of a positive anti-smoking approach after myocardial infarction. A detailed explanation accompanied by very firm advice to stop smoking in hospital was followed up at a special clinic and reinforced by a visit from a health visitor to the home, with advice being extended to the family. This resulted in 63.2 per cent remaining abstinent for 1 to 3 years while over half of the remainder decreased their cigarette consumption considerably. This compares with only 27.5 per cent ceasing in the control group who had received conventional advice but who had not been exposed to this intensive approach.[11]

Of the sixty-four smokers in our series, six said that they had been given no advice regarding smoking in hospital, these all being cigarette smokers. Twenty-five said that they had been given no advice regarding smoking by general practitioners, and four claimed that no advice regarding smoking had been given to them by either hospital or general practitioner. The possibilities are either that advice was given and the patients forgot, that it was given but not effectively communicated to the patients or that it was not given at all. Some remarked that the doctor himself smoked and they assumed that this was the reason why he did not advise them. This was said more often about general practitioners — only one patient referred to a hospital doctor smoking (which may partly be because the smoking habits of hospital doctors were less visible to patients). Of the four patients claiming no advice at all, one stopped, one changed to pipe smoking, one reduced from 30 to 20 cigarettes a day and one remained the same, at 30 a day.

The advice to patients was categorised with regard to how emphatic it was to stop, whether change to pipe or cigars was mentioned, and whether there was discrepancy in advice between hospital and general practitioner, but no significant statistical difference was found when these criteria were compared.

Several studies have noted that older smokers are likely to be more successful in stopping than are younger ones.[12, 13, 14] In this series men aged over 45 were much more successful than the youngest age group of whom only 8 per cent stopped, although, among those over 45, the intermediate age groups had a higher success rate (nearly one half) than those aged over 55 (under one third) where some tended to cut down consumption rather than to stop entirely. It is often suggested that older people are more concerned about their health and thus more likely to follow advice which they feel will reduce the chance of further illness.

Among men in this series who neither stopped nor cut down were two who had previously been strongly advised to do so on account of coexisting chest conditions. Only two men were referred to anti-smoking clinics and only one of these attended. Having previously smoked 80 cigarettes a day, he resumed smoking a few daily in convalescent hospital and, at six months, following attendance at the anti-smoking clinic, was smoking 20 a day.

Altogether, 63 per cent of smokers had stopped smoking at discharge from hospital but the number had fallen to 38 per cent at three months and 34 per cent at six months, that is, to a level very similar to the rate achieved in the ordinary Dundee anti-smoking clinics (33.6 per cent), six months after beginning attendance. It is also much closer to the rate reached by the controls among the Edinburgh myocardial infarction population (27.5 per cent) at 12 to 36 months) than to that achieved by the Edinburgh patients who received intensive advice and sustained follow-up (63.2 per cent).

Husband-Wife Interaction in Smoking Habits

We were particularly interested in the social characteristics of men who were still heavy smokers a year after infarction as compared with the characteristics of men who either were non-smokers at infarction or who stopped smoking after infarction and how these related both to wives' predictions and to wives' own smoking habits. For interviews we used the categories recommended by the Medical Research Council[15] but to simplify the complex data we are here describing those in MRC categories 2 and 3 (1-14 cigarettes or equivalent per day) as moderate smokers; and those in MRC categories 4 and 5 (15-24 and 25+ respectively) as heavy smokers.

Both at infarction and a year later there were some very minor differences between wives' reports of husbands' smoking habits and the men's own reports, eight husbands describing their smoking in terms which put them one category lower than that chosen by their wives; this included three men who considered themselves as non-smokers, although on their wives' report, they would have been considered as coming within MRC smoking category 2 (1-4 cigarettes per day). In the following section we use the wives' reports.

At infarction three men out of every four were heavy smokers and only one in every eight was a non-smoker. Compared with non-manual men, higher proportions of manual workers were heavy smokers and fewer were non-smokers. Younger men were more often heavy smokers than older men and among the 13 men aged under 44, 12 were heavy smokers and none was a non-smoker (Table 9.4).

One woman in every four was a heavy smoker (distribution ranging from fewer than one out of every five, among women married to non-manual workers, to nearly one third among those married to manual workers). Higher proportions were non-smokers — three out of every five non-manual women and two out of every five manual women. Women aged over 55 were seldom heavy smokers

(Table 9.5).

So far, we have seen that in smoking habits at infarction manual workers were more often at a disadvantage than non-manual workers (fewer non-smokers, more heavy smokers, fewer non-smoking and more heavy smoking wives) and younger men more often at a disadvantage compared with older men.

One year later, nearly one third of the men who were smokers at infarction had stopped, thus bringing the total of non-smokers to over two out of every five; nevertheless over one quarter were still in the two heaviest categories (Table 9.6). Over one half of the non-manual men were now non-smokers compared with just over one third of the manual workers, the difference between them having widened. At the other extreme only one in every ten of the non-manual workers was still a heavy smoker compared with nearly two in every five manual workers, so in this respect too the gap between social class groupings had widened. While half the men of intermediate age were now non-smokers and nearly as many older men, fewer than one in six of the youngest men had stopped.

Overall, then, differences favouring non-manual workers and men aged over 45 had increased in the course of the post-infarction career.

Comparison of other social characteristics of the 21 persistent heavy smokers with the rest of the series, and particularly with 32 men who had either been non-smokers before infarction or had become so since, showed a number of other respects in which persistent heavy smokers were disadvantaged; nearly all of these however, correlated with the different social class composition of the groups; for instance, persistent heavy smokers more often had fathers who had been in less skilled occupations and they were also more often married to women who had been in less skilled occupations.

As we have seen in Chapter 6, wives were asked while their husbands were in hospital what they thought their husbands would do about smoking. Some said 'He *has* stopped now', i.e. while in hospital, but on closer questioning, did not expect this to last. Twenty wives were, however, very confident and their confidence appeared justified since 16 of their husbands, that is four out of every five, became non-smokers and none was a heavy smoker a year later. A considerably larger number of women (34) had, however, been very pessimistic or uncertain and only six of their husbands fewer than one in every five became non-smokers while two in every five remained heavy smokers. Men whose wives had thought that they might cut down were more often in the heavy categories (Table 9.7).

We also wondered how wives' smoking habits were related to their husbands' habits before infarction and to subsequent changes by both of them. One way of looking at the rather complex picture is to compare the 35 women who were non-smokers at first interview with the 20 women who were heavy smokers. At that time nearly three quarters of the non-smoking women were married to heavy smokers and fewer than one in every five non-smokers had non-smoking husbands; however, one year later, considerable improvement in their husbands' smoking patterns had occurred, nearly half now being non-smokers and only one quarter still being heavy smokers (Table 9.8).

In contrast, 17 men married to women who were heavy smokers at first interview were themselves heavy smokers at that time while the remaining three were in the moderate category: a year later, only four of these 20 men had become non-smokers and eight were still heavy smokers. This seems to suggest that wives' pre-infarction smoking habits may be important in influencing their husbands' adaptation to post-infarction advice on smoking.

Overall (as already shown in Table 9.5), the level of change among women themselves was lower, partly because nearly half of them were already non-smokers and so there was less scope for change than existed among the men. Seven women reported stopping after husband's infarction, all but one of these previously being moderate smokers; among their husbands two men were already non-smokers, three became non-smokers, one decreased and one remained in the same category. Three other women decreased from a heavy to a moderate category, but only one of their husbands stopped, the other two remaining heavy smokers. So it seems that in this series change in womens' smoking habits was rather less important than their habits before their husbands' illness. (As we note in Chapter 13, three wives were later found to have died in the interval between 12 months and four years; all had been heavy smokers at first interview and had not stopped at second interview.)

In the reverse direction, there were instances of some women starting, resuming or increasing smoking after their husbands' infarction. Three women who had been non-smokers at first interview began, or resumed, smoking while husbands were in hospital and three more increased from a moderate to a heavy category. A few others increased slightly although not to the extent of moving into a separate category.

Apart from one former non-smoker who said she had started

smoking to compensate for keeping to a diet after joining a slimming club all the other women who had started or increased smoking during the year attributed this to worry arising from their husbands' illness. A previous heavy smoker admitted 'I'm smoking too many, about 20 a day, but it doesn't seem to bother him and I don't smoke in the bedroom.'

When women were asked about their own smoking habits at first interview, they were deliberately not asked whether they intended to make changes. However, many spontaneously made comments at both interviews linking their own and their husbands' smoking habits. One woman who doubted if her husband could stop explained 'He's like me, I can give up for three months, but I put on so much weight, I have to start again. He's the same.' Several said that husbands had been trying to stop before infarction and some women had been trying also.

One couple had stopped and started again several times and, shortly before infarction, the husband had sent away for a 'smoking cure' (a mouth wash type of preparation) for both of them, which he had been trying out (and very much disliking) on the day before infarction. His wife said that their efforts had been both on health and financial grounds but principally the former (lung cancer rather than heart disease having been seen as the risk); she and their son were determined to stop when he came home. Another woman said that she had stopped several years previously after herself having a heart attack. Her husband and children tried to stop at that time and refrained from smoking when in the same room as her but continued smoking upstairs.

Another couple had stopped successfully several years before; this woman explained 'It was at the time of the cancer scare and also to save money. It's no good one of you stopping so I stopped when he did. And, of course, if I had been smoking, I'd have been smoking *more* now.' Several said they would stop when their husbands came home — 'to continue wouldna be fair to him', 'I wouldna be so cruel', 'it would be a temptation to him', although one or two thought they might smoke in secret when husbands were not at home.

One woman appeared very aware of the process of interaction, past and present, explaining

He's pretty determined to stop, after listening to them coughing and gasping for breath in the ward at night. I really think he will, *if I do.* I *had* stopped once for six months and he started me off again — I don't know if it was him leaving ash and ends round the house — so I'll stop in case I start him off. But don't tell my

mother — though I've a grown-up son I don't like my mother to
know about my smoking.

Both she and her husband in fact stopped and she reported a year
later; 'He *does* find it hard at work because the men smoke there, but
he doesn't take any at all. I stopped to help him because I know how
hard it is to stop alone.' She added

> I was supposed to stop after an operation several years ago and I
> used to blame him for starting me off again, though I know I
> should have blamed my lack of willpower, so I knew this time I
> *had* to stop — I'd said before that it was easy for the doctor to say
> I should stop when he [the doctor] didn't smoke, but, truthfully,
> I must say that it's only now since I gave up smoking to help my
> husband that I've felt the good of my own operation.

Another woman said 'He was told to stop and stopped at once. I
thought I would be better to stop too. It was difficult for a bit but
it doesn't worry me now. If I'd kept on it would have put him in the
mood for it too.' Some women who stopped or cut down
explained this as on account of their own health or because they could
no longer afford to smoke.

Absence of Compensatory Roles

When women described their husbands' reluctance or inability to
abandon the role of smoker there was often an underlying assumption
that there were few or no other positive roles available to them. We
have seen in the preceding chapter that many men felt that their work
roles were under threat and many women saw these work roles as
central to their husbands' self-concepts. There were indications, cited
in this and the following chapter, of a feeling of loss or diminution in
other roles which may have increased the tendency to cling all the
more to the smoking role, especially since abandoning the habit of
offering and accepting cigarettes may mean withdrawal from the
customary satisfactions of participating in a social exchange, instead
setting oneself apart from, and perhaps seeming to become less
acceptable to, other members of the social network.

In pilot interviews a phrase which had frequently occurred was
the definition of a heart attack as being a warning or a lesson. When
wives of men in this series were asked at second interviews what they
thought this meant, some saw it in positive terms as a lesson to be

learned not only for their husbands but also for themselves, 'It's been a great lesson to us all to change our way of life, especially diet and exercise', said one with the implication that learning a lesson added something to the self-concept of each member of the family. Among others, however, it was often taken in more negative terms as a warning: 'It's a warning to take it easy — he says he was lucky, some people don't get one', 'It's your heart crying out to slow down — if you don't take things easier, graver things may happen.' One woman made a distinction 'It's possibly a warning to slow down, but it's not a lesson unless you take heed and he hasna.'

Many women appeared to perceive husbands as previously having been very strongly committed to instrumental roles both in work settings and social networks ('He feels the factory will fall down without him', 'I think they play on him a bit at work', 'The neighbours come to him when they want something done'). Such activities had been reduced after the illness, although there were occasional indications that withdrawal from instrumental roles might be more easily accepted by neighbours ('I think they don't like to bother him the same as before') than by employers ('They seem to be on at him to do overtime more than before') or by close kin ('His mother still thinks he should do her decorating').

Activities increased or taken up as a result of the illness were, especially among manual workers, seldom of a kind that appeared to give any compensatory sense of role gain. Walking, where continued as a regular activity, was generally solitary, although one factory worker had found fortuitously a workmate following similar health advice with whom he shared lunch hour walks in a nearby park. Like another manual worker, cited earlier, who on taking up golf, was joined by his son and son-in-law, he was an exception in finding outdoor companionship. Men who had not returned to work and who had taken on wives' household tasks appeared to derive some satisfaction thereby but seldom sufficient to balance the satisfactions derived from conventional work role.

This absence of compensatory roles and activities seemed the sadder because most often men's intense commitment to instrumental roles appeared to have been accompanied by a deficiency in respect of expressive roles. Here, a limited amount of change could be seen, some men being said by their wives to have become more 'open' and 'considerate' since the illness and sometimes the experience was described as having brought them closer to wives and families. Occasionally there were indications that family understanding resulting from the illness had enhanced self-esteem — 'He knows he's valued for himself', 'He felt that we were pulling with him' — sometimes with the implication that some might have lacked such self-esteem before the illness.

Sometimes, insight and initiative by wives could be seen making it easier for men to accept the change of values required when the demands of a health career must take precedence over an occupational career, as in a family where the wife explained that her husband's work as a supervisor 'meant responsibility and tension and it was heavy because he was always mucking in with the men though he shouldna, so I put it to him that he's too much to do and, even if it's less money, lighter work would be better for him, so that's when he went to see his boss and volunteered for demotion'. All too often, however, the negotiation of such role transitions appeared beset by unexpressed anxieties and uncertainties.

We wondered to what extent rearrangements in roles and changes in self-concepts among the men might be conducive to changed roles and perceptions among their wives. The next chapter draws upon the wives' perceptions at twelve months of the effects on everyday family life.

Notes

1. Goffman, E. (1962). On Cooling the Mark Out: Some Aspects of Adaptation to Failure. In: Rose, A.M. (ed.) *Human Behavior and Social Processes*, London, Routledge and Kegan Paul.
2. Garrity, T.F. (1973). Vocational Adjustment After First Myocardial Infarction: Comparative Assessment of Several Variables Suggested in the Literature. *Social Science and Medicine* 7, 705-17.
3. Wishnie, H.A., Hackett, T.P. and Cassem, N.H. (1971). Psychological Hazards of Convalescence Following Myocardial Infarction. *Journal of the American Medical Association* 215, 1292-6
4. Monteiro, L.A. (1973). After Heart Attack: Behavioral Expectations for the Cardiac. *Social Science and Medicine* 7, 555-65.
5. Royal College of Physicians (1971). *Smoking and Health Now*, London, Pitman Medical.
6. Russell, M.A.H. (1971). Cigarette Dependence: I Nature and Classification and II Doctor's Role in Management. *British Medical Journal* 2, 330-31 and 393-5.
7. McKennell, A.C. and Thomas, R.K. (1967). *Adults' and Adolescents' Smoking Habits and Attitudes*, Government Social Survey Report, London, HMSO.
8. Royal College of Physicians (1962). *Smoking and Health*, London, Pitman Medical.
9. Fee, W.M. and Benson, C. (1971). Group Therapy: A Review of 6 Years' Experience in a Scottish Anti-Smoking Clinic. *Community Medicine* 126, 361-4.
10. Graham S. and Gibson, R.W. (1971). Cessation of Patterned Behaviour: Withdrawal from Smoking. *Social Science and Medicine* 5, 319-37.

11. Burt, A., Illingworth, D., Shaw, T.R.D., Thornley P., White, P. and Turner, R. (1974). Stopping Smoking After Myocardial Infarction. *Lancet* 1, 304-6.
12. Hammond, E.C. and Garfinkel, L. (1964). Changes in Cigarette Smoking. *Journal of the National Cancer Institute* 33, 49-64.
13. Todd, G.F. (1969). *Statistics of Smoking in the United Kingdom*. Research Paper No.1, 5th ed, London, Tobacco Research Council. Table 54.
14. Eisinger, R.S. (1971). Psychosocial Predictors of Smoking Recidivism. *Journal of Health and Social Behaviour* 12, 355-62.
15. Medical Research Council (1966). *Questionnaire on Respiratory Symptoms*. Dawlish, W.J. Holman.

10 IMPACT ON EVERYDAY FAMILY LIFE: WIVES' VIEWS

One might have expected that the sense of role loss among men which has been indicated in the preceding chapters would evoke a sense of role gain among wives. This seemed to be so to a limited degree only. Accustomed as they were to making continual minor adjustments to the combined demands of husbands, children and kin, most women seemed to view the taking on of extra burdens and responsibilities as an intrinsic and inevitable part of their existing roles, rather than as amounting to a change of role or a different way of life. They appeared to feel that the little which they could do was insignificant compared with adverse factors in the personality, health or work setting of their husbands which 'nobody can alter'.

Never the less, a great deal of minor change had in fact taken place and we wanted to document something of the impact on everyday family life, especially the kind of changes which wives found hard to make and the type of practical and emotional support which they considered had come from professional services and from the informal resources of their social networks. We had it in mind that, as Mechanic has written,

> Illness behaviour and reactions to the ill are aspects of a coping dialogue in which the active participants are often actively striving to meet their responsibilities, to control their environment, and to make everyday circumstances more tolerable and predictable. It is these active strivings — the stuff of human behaviour — which are often neglected and ignored in many behavioural science theories that view human behaviour as fixed and inflexible, rather than as continuously changing in response to environmental demands and challenges.[1]

It is not easy to make meaningful comparisons between different families because life-styles and definitions of what is normal varied so widely, as did women's perception of both the need and the scope for change. It proved possible, never the less, to explore some areas in which wives' roles and perceptions seemed particularly important. Many differences which emerged appeared to be associated with social class and/or age and they are discussed here; some which appeared, additionally, to have an association with outcome are discussed further in the following chapter.

The health of the women themselves was clearly of importance since, as Chapter 5 has illustrated, many had been suffering during the pre-infarction career from conditions likely to cause concern within the family and possibly to divert attention from their husbands' symptoms. Comparison of the post-infarction year with the preceding one showed the number of women consulting general practitioners to be remarkably constant, again just under two thirds. These were not always the same women; never the less the difference between classes remained much as before, three out of every four wives of skilled manual workers seeking medical advice compared with only half the non-manual wives and just over half the wives of less skilled workers.

As we have seen in Chapter 5, there had been in the pre-infarction year no consistent difference in women's consultation rate with wife's age and little with husband's age. This continued to be true during the post-infarction year in respect of wife's age but differences did appear in respect of husband's age, wives of men aged under 45 and over 54 more often reporting consultations on their own behalf. Since men in these two age groups less often had favourable outcomes than did those of intermediate age (as will be seen in Chapter 11), this may suggest some degree of interaction between the health status of the spouses (Table 10.1).

During the year following husbands' illness, ten of the women were admitted to hospital as inpatients (the same as in the preceding year), including two who had been awaiting admission at the time of husbands' illness, and two of those who had been inpatients in the previous year, as well as one who had been attending as an outpatient. Three of the ten were admitted for gynaecological operations and four required other operations. One woman was admitted on account of two small heart attacks, one because of severe angina and one because of a 'nervous breakdown'. Two more women were awaiting admission for hysterectomy. Nine women had attended outpatient clinics for investigation and treatment (one of these had been an inpatient and two, outpatients, in the previous year). Those who consulted general practitioners only, mentioned conditions of varying degrees of severity, some long-term and others which, they claimed, were attributed by their doctors to reactions to their husbands' illness.

Apart from their health we had wondered if women's work roles would change following infarction. As indicated in Chapter 6 they did

not themselves think this would happen and they proved to be
correct, such changes as occurred being relatively minor. Among
non-manual wives, five, or less than one quarter, made some changes.
One woman, who worked with her self-employed husband in a
marginally viable business, increased her hours of work 'in order to
spare him'. However, a second woman, also working with her husband
in self-employment, reversed this pattern by reducing her hours with
the intention of thereby discouraging him from taking on extra
work. In contrast to the previous couple, they had a thriving
business, employees and more 'room for manoeuvre'. Another two
women married to non-manual men changed their hours of employment
to give more time to their husbands and one changed her job only
when she was made redundant.

Meanwhile, among manual workers' wives none of the six women
who were unemployed or off work owing to illness at first interview had
returned to work and two more women were now off work for
health reasons. Two full-time workers had changed jobs after
redundancy but were doing the same hours. One childless non-working
wife had begun full-time work (her husband had previously objected to
her working).

In general, their husbands' illness appeared to make little long-term
impact on wives' working roles and many reported that, quite apart
from the reassurance provided by having a second income, going to
work helped to keep them from worrying excessively. These findings
were in accordance with those of Skelton and Dominian[2] whose series
of 65 wives was of comparable age and social class. Like them, when
speculating on possible effects if men were treated at home rather than
in hospital, we were very aware that this could create considerable
difficulties for working wives, which would need to be taken into
account before any changes in this direction might be made.

It will be asked whether wives going out to work contributed to
difficulties in the husbands' post-infarction career. The evidence,
which is discussed more fully in Chapter 11, did not seem to suggest
this and, as at first interview, working wives often referred to their
jobs as a reason why they did not need to worry unduly about money
when their husbands were ill. As had been found among women in an
Aberdeen survey[3] the type of work and the hours which women were
prepared to do were chosen to fit in with the needs of their families
as they saw these and, although some of them operated on a very tight
timetable, the general level of housekeeping noted at interviews
appeared high. Some of the non-working wives would have liked to

take on outside work and spoke of feeling this more strongly as the
result of their husbands' illness but were unable to do so either because
husbands objected or because there were no suitable opportunities.

Among domestic changes one which was reported by over half the
women was in respect of the kind of food which they gave their
husbands and/or the way of preparing it. The proportion decreased
with social class from two thirds of wives of men in Social Classes I
and II to under half of the women married to less skilled workers,
who more often mentioned the cost of suitable foods as a difficulty.
Wives of men in the intermediate age groups more often reported
making changes in food than did wives of youngest and oldest men
(Table 10.2).

Changes were generally in the direction of increased consumption
of vegetables and fish with decrease in fats and starch and the
substitution of grilling for frying (one woman said that she had
thrown away her frying pan). A few women claimed that their
previous diet had been of the kind suggested: this was generally
because the husband had already been under medical care or because
either he or his wife had been slimming. Thirteen women reported
finding the changes difficult to make, non-manual wives saying this
relatively more often than other women. Some were concerned about
making the food acceptable to their husbands, some about the effect
on the rest of the family while others were uncertain about the safety
of certain foods, particularly eggs.

We had wondered whether the illness might be seen as causing
financial worries. At first interview, women had been asked if they
thought that money would be a big problem during recovery. One in
every five was emphatic that it would be and a further one in five
thought it might be to some extent. At second interview there was
only a slight increase in those who had found money a major problem.
As one would expect, there was a steep gradient with social class,
four out of every five of women married to men in classes I and II
saying that it had not been a problem at all, compared with under
one third in classes IV and V. Working wives often referred to their
own jobs as a reason for not needing to worry, or to worry so much,
about money. Two non-manual wives who shared marginal self-
employment with husbands were very worried; the husband of one
was not back at work, the other was working but was seen by his
wife as still very much affected, both by the illness and by their
business difficulties. (It should be remembered that these interviews
took place at a time when worries about inflation had not yet become

'normal', Table 10.2).

Approximately half the women said that they felt they had more general responsibilities since their husbands' illness, for instance in regard to finance, the children or planning for the future, but some said that, as they had always taken a large share of responsibilities, the illness had not made much difference. One woman explained that this was because her husband's parents had died young so that he hadn't had much experience of home life, 'Not', she added 'that I decide things over his head, we work it out together but I've often to *start* things.' Other women took the view that it was best not to remove responsibilities for more than the first few weeks lest this should be bad for self-respect: 'I let him take over again — I wouldn't take his responsibilities from him' (see Table 10.2).

Although several husbands were reported as not having been accustomed before the illness to undertaking any household tasks, nearly three out of every four women reported that some one (usually herself and frequently in co-operation with children) had taken over some tasks from husbands and in most cases this rearrangement was still in force twelve months after the illness. For instance, although the husband might have resumed weeding the garden, the wife or a son would cut the grass. Sometimes neighbours were mentioned as helping with gardening, but generally this had been in the early stages only. Women married to young manual workers least often reported the taking over of household tasks. This, however, is an area in which change is not only intricately tied up both with life-style before infarction but also with the outcome of the illness and is discussed further in relation to outcome in the following chapter (see Table 10.2).

At first interview questions had not been included specifically on sexual intercourse; there were however indications, expressed particularly by younger wives but perhaps implicit in the more general worries of others, of considerable anxiety lest intercourse should precipitate pain or another infarction. A labourer's wife said that she was very worried 'if he will be able and if it would be bad for him', adding that the first thing he had said when she went to see him in hospital was 'You know what this means — I'm no' a man any more.' There was little evidence of wives having received reassurance or advice from medical services and since it was mainly the younger wives who expressed concern, this appears to be an area in which counselling will increasingly be needed from the very beginning of the post-infarction career both by men and their wives.

At second interview, provided that children or others were not present, women were asked if frequency of intercourse had remained the same or had increased or decreased since the illness. Of the 41 women who were asked this, one reported intercourse to be more frequent. Of the remainder, one third considered frequency to be about the same while two thirds reported a decrease. Among the latter there was a steep gradient with age, women aged over 55 often adding that they considered reduced frequency to be normal for their age and that of their husbands and not necessarily related to the illness (Table 10.2). This, like the indications of anxiety about deciding when intercourse could safely be resumed, is in accordance with the findings of Skelton and Dominian whose series was of comparable age. Although the level of anxiety appeared high, there was very little evidence of advice having been sought from or offered by, medical services.

Approximately two out of every three women considered that some kind of personality change had occurred in their husbands since the illness, although a few thought such changes had been only temporary (Table 10.2). Those married to men of intermediate age thought this more often than did others. As Skelton and Dominian found, changes were generally in the direction of men being thought more irritable and dependent; however, occasionally, men were described as becoming more considerate and better tempered. Exceptionally, also, some were said to have become more 'open'. More often, however, they were described as still 'bottling things up' or 'keeping them to themselves'. Overall, nearly half the women described their husbands as being very reluctant to confide in them or to discuss worries, this proportion being highest among wives of less skilled workers and men aged under 44 and lowest among women married to men in Social Classes I and II (Table 10.2).

Many women considered that the worst aspect of the illness for their husbands was not being able to do all that they could before. Some men and their wives spoke of the illness as constituting a lesson or a warning to change their way of life but this recognition did not necessarily mean that all the implications were accepted. A manual worker's wife explained: 'He says it was a warning to slow down and not do things you can when you're younger – he doesn't mind admitting that we are getting older.' Later however, she added: 'He does get annoyed if he feels people are looking at him when it's me carrying the heavy shopping instead of him.' Similarly it might not be too difficult for a man to accept help from old friends at work but less easy when it meant, for instance, explaining to a new workmate why he should not lift a heavy load. Particularly because many men looked as though they were 'back to normal', they were exposed to a lack of congruence between the new definitions which they had been compelled to accept and those which they expected would be made by casual onlookers or new acquaintances. Such situations appeared particularly likely to face manual workers partly because of the nature of their work and family life-style but also because members of their social networks seemed less often to be experienced and tactful in recognising and handling the delicate role transformations involved. (This latter point is further considered in Chapters 11 and 12.)

At first interview many women had seemed to see their husbands as trapped in some kind of complex interaction between their personalities and their work or social situation. These conditions were felt still to obtain twelve months later. Referring back to what they now thought might have caused their husbands' illness, many women again named more than one factor, two out of every three indicating some aspect of personality, a slightly smaller number naming work and half mentioning other reasons, including previous ill-health, heredity, overweight, smoking and problems in family or wider network. Non-manual women more often mentioned a combination of personality and work factors, while wives of manual workers more often spoke of the combined effect of personality and other factors.

When asked about husbands' work since the illness, half the women whose husbands were back at work at twelve months considered that there had been change in work habits, wives of non-manual workers and men in intermediate age groups thinking this more often than others (Table 10.2).

Many women were worried about the possibility of recurrence of the illness, a common experience being rapidly rising anxiety if men were late in coming home. Approximately one in every four women thought that their husbands also worried about recurrence, although an equal number thought that they did not. The remaining half did not know, this high proportion reflecting the feeling, described earlier, that many husbands did not confide in them (Table 10.2).

Wives' Perception of Communication with Doctors

Mechanic has emphasised that doctors and patients 'often operate within quite different assumptive worlds and often lack awareness of the extent to which their assumptions are different'. Some women, like the one described in Chapter 6, who distinguished between her attitude to doctors moulded during service in a doctor's household and her husband's attitude shaped by his mother's distrust of the profession, seemed explicitly or implicitly aware of the gap and — in varying degree — felt that they had a role in trying to bridge it.

Asked whether their husbands had talked to general practitioners about their illness as much as they, the wives, thought they should, just over half replied affirmatively — rather fewer than had expected this would happen (Table 10.2). Some women mentioned situational factors which had contributed to reducing contact with doctors. For instance, two families had moved house in order to cut down on the time that men spent in travelling to work and thus had to find new doctors, while in another case the general practitioner retired. These men were all seen as reluctant to contact new doctors, let alone discuss health problems with them.

For some other men, the doctor's role as diagnostician and adviser appeared to be seen as secondary to his role as gatekeeper to employment. An extremely conscientious tradesman had a second attack one evening soon after returning to work, but, although in great pain, refused to let his wife call the doctor until morning. She explained 'It's not the fear of the doctor or going to hospital, it's the idea of having to stay off work. "If I get the doctor I'll be off again" he says.'

The wife of a self-employed man who had earlier hoped that her husband's attitude would change said

Well, sometimes he doesn't tell the doctor — I generally go in with him and sometimes I tell the doctor because my husband thinks it's perhaps trivial — it's his first illness and he's never been used to telling the doctor things and he doesn't want to bother him, and of course he never liked the thought of being off work, so all these things make him backward at talking to the doctor. At one stage, perhaps around six months ago, he was taking a turn every night of the week and I got him to go to the doctor then — before that it was happening just two nights in the week and he wouldn't go — it wasn't anything, he said then, to bother the doctor with.

In such instances there appeared to be lack of congruence between the definitions of husband and wife as to when symptoms were serious enough to take priority over competing motivations. Although Skelton and Dominian do not specifically refer to differences between husbands and wives in this respect, they also found evidence of great anxiety among wives as to whether medical aid or reassurance was needed when chest pain occurred as it did in the great majority of cases in their series. In our series, uncertainty among wives as to what was the right action to take resulted in a great deal of role strain.

Where communication between doctor and patient is felt to be inadequate the role of lay consultants becomes correspondingly important. An example of how this process may work was provided by a very articulate woman who herself suffered two small heart attacks during the course of her husband's post-infarction career and who was very satisfied with the explanation given to her, which she contrasted with the lack of advice offered to her husband. She said,

> He wasn't told much except about smoking — in fact he was a bit disappointed, he was not told what his limitations were and what he could do. I know you're supposed to find out for yourself but you might do something beyond your limitations because you don't know. I got a lot of advice. He was not told anything like that. I've been able to hand on some of my advice to him. The doctor at the hospital explained what caused my heart attacks. I would have worried but he gave me plenty of time to ask questions and explained that the failure was only temporary. If he hadn't told me I would have gone home worrying. It was a great help and reassured me — I had quite a different attitude from my husband. It's not as though he hadn't had a serious attack, more serious than mine, but I got the better advice.

Women were also asked if they had themselves talked to their husband's general practitioner about his illness. Five wives said they had done so only at the time of hospitalisation, and if they are included, two out of every five had done so. Generally the talks appeared to have taken place in a fairly fortuitous manner, when the woman was showing the doctor out, when she met him in the street or when she was consulting him on her own behalf. But, since women married to non-manual workers in Social Class IIIa and women married to less skilled workers reported this slightly more often, and since women in these groups were also more often dissatisfied with their husband's consulting habits, it may be that some had manufactured the opportunity to talk to the doctor (Table 10.2).

Occasionally talks had taken place at the doctor's instigation, and a few women seemed to feel caught in a conflict between their own inability to influence their husband's behaviour and the doctor's

expectation that they could and should do so. For instance, a
labourer's wife explained,

> When I was up at the doctor's last week with the wee lass he said
> he was glad to see me because my husband *has* to stop smoking and
> overeating — the fat is lying on the heart — but the problem is I
> can't get him to. I don't know whether the doctor told him how
> serious it is or whether I'm meant to. I've been feeling all tensed
> up since the doctor told me — my stomach was churning round and
> round . . . I think the doctor was thinking I'd make him give up
> smoking and cut down on food but I don't seem to know how to.
> You know how it is when you're trying to take in what the
> doctor's telling you — you can't find words to ask him how you're
> to do it.

At the other extreme, some wives, especially those who defined the
illness as now over, said that they had felt no need to talk to the
doctor themselves because they were quite confident that everything
had been discussed adequately and their husbands had passed on to
them all the information obtained from the doctor.

As Mechanic has emphasised, patients and doctors who share
particular cultural traits relate to one another more easily. These latter
women were more often married to men in non-manual occupations
and both spouses more often shared a common frame of reference
with their doctors. They were also more often women who confided in
and were confided in by their husbands.

Medical Regimens

A study by Milton Davis[4] has suggested that in the USA at least one
third of patients disregard doctors' advice. He related this to deviant
communication between doctor and patient, difficulties in
communication and attempts by doctors and patients to control each
other.

Overall in this series, two out of every three wives said they
thought that such advice as husbands had been given was practicable.
There is some slight evidence that women married to men in minor
non-manual occupations such as clerks and salesmen as well as those
married to men in less skilled occupations less often thought this, but
it must be remembered that numbers in these classes represented in
this series are very small. There are, however, bigger differences with
age of husband — a gradient showing the proportion of women who

thought the advice practicable increasing from half among those married to men under 44 to three quarters of those with husbands aged over 55 (Table 10.2).

When asked whether husbands, in fact, followed such advice, half the women thought that their husbands kept to it all, and seven women said they kept to none of it (Table 10.2). The discrepancy between the answers to this and to the previous question was summed up by one woman who said that the advice was practicable enough — *'but not for him'.* Smoking was often mentioned in this context as something that husbands had not been able to adjust, and difficulty in changing or maintaining changed work habits was also to the fore in women's comments, for instance heavy lifting by van drivers. Women explained: 'He's always been used to being independent', 'He says you canna always be asking your mates for help.'

Looking at class differences on this question and the previous one, the proportions of women married to men in non-manual occupations corresponded closely with those answering the previous question affirmatively. The percentages for the wives of manual workers were much lower, however, lack of cungruence with the previous question being particularly marked for skilled workers. This may to some extent reflect a difference between this group and the less skilled workers in that relatively more of the latter were already accustomed to living with adversity or illness and so perhaps their perception of what was practicable was closer to reality.

The age pattern for this question showed a very sharp difference between the very youngest men and all others, for only one woman married to a man in this age group thought that her husband followed all advice, in contrast to women married to men in the older age groups in which over half the wives reported this. Although numbers are small, these young men seem a very vulnerable category and this is reflected in the fact that only half of them were back at work after a year. They were also heavily biassed towards manual work and local origin. Only one was in Social Class II and two in Social Class IIIa (non-manual) while only one was not local in origin. Of the seven women who said that their husbands kept to no advice at all, six were married to manual workers and six to men in the two younger age groups, that is men aged under 49.

Mechanic suggests that compliance with medical advice 'appears to be facilitated by family harmony and stability, as the patient is more likely to receive help and encouragement in adopting new patterns under such circumstances'. On the assumption that the

adoption of either an extremely authoritarian role or an extremely
negative or unco-operative role by wives would be disadvantageous,
the women were asked if they had needed to remind husbands much
about keeping to advice and their answers were grouped into three
types of response. At one extreme there were answers indicating that
women felt they took a great deal of positive or active responsibility
for this. Overall, one woman in every five gave this type of answer.
At the other extreme, nine women, or one in every eight, gave answers
which were predominantly negative, such as 'I've given up trying',
'he wouldna heed me', 'It's no use'. In between these two extremes
one third said they did not need to remind husbands or thought it
better not do so and another one third said they only reminded
them occasionally. Combining these two gives just over two thirds
playing, as they seemed to see it, a moderate role (Table 10.2).

Again there are differences by age and class, women married to
men in Social Class III (in this instance, wives of men with clerical and
supervisory jobs from IIIa converging with the wives of skilled manual
workers) more often giving answers indicating an extreme or very
positive role. Four out of every five of women married to men in
Social Classes I and II appeared to adopt a moderate role which
seems congruent with their account of husbands keeping to all
advice, but women married to less skilled workers appeared
equally often to keep to a moderate role although reporting that
their husbands could not keep to all advice. It might be more
appropriate to consider these latter women as being forced by
overwhelming difficulties into playing a passive role rather than as
adopting a moderate role. Some of them were, indeed, conscious of
the situation in which they felt trapped. As the wife of a farm worker
put it, 'I've had to forget about the smoking because I found arguing
about it did more harm than the smoking. I felt I was turning into
a nag.' She added 'It would be better if the doctor would tell him
but he would need to keep at it. He did tell him *once*.'

In terms of age more than two out of every three women married
to men in the intermediate age groups gave answers suggesting a
moderate role, while only half the women married to men in the
youngest age group did so, and women married to men in the
oldest age group have the next lowest rate. Of the two extreme types
of responses, women married to the youngest men appeared more
often to give the negative 'He wouldna heed me' type of answer and
women married to the older men more often gave answers indicating
an active or positive, protective role.

Comments made by women when enlarging on these and other questions which point in similar directions seemed to indicate a pattern in which wives of men in Social Classes I and II more often were reasonably content with their husbands' adaptation. Relatively more of them seemed to feel that their husbands had 'room to manoeuvre' both in terms of situation and personality. The accounts given by wives in other social classes seemed more often to indicate men trapped either by psychological or by situational difficulties — and frequently both. Youngest men also appeared vulnerable in both respects.

It would not be realistic to ignore the fact that something of a stereotype appears to exist both in the minds of many members of the medical profession and the public generally indicting 'nagging wives' as at least a contributory factor to heart disease in men and a possible hindrance to recovery. We have seen that a small minority of women perceived themselves as having to take a very positive or extreme role in their husbands' post-infarction regimen, which might be interpreted as 'nagging' while others appeared conscious of the dangers of this role and anxious to avoid it.

This does not exclude the possibility that 'nagging' might never the less have occurred. To isolate it, however, as a causal factor or as a hindrance to recovery seems, however, a rather simplistic view which underestimates the complexity of family interaction. Our evidence suggests rather that, although wives were less often inhibited in expressive roles than were their husbands, in many families both partners lacked in varying degrees the interpersonal skills which facilitate coping with role change. Such skills would have made it easier to meet the changes which they were facing in family and work settings before the illness and would also have facilitated renegotiation of roles in the post-infarction career.[5]

Some wives did mention making changes in their own expressive roles and sometimes these indicated a reordering of experience to the extent of recognising previous behaviours as detrimental: 'I'm perhaps a bit more considerate. Before, when he came home, I might say that such and such needed doing in the house or garden and he'd do it and go on and on at it.' Other women indicated that they tried to be tactful and to think before they said anything that might worry husbands; sometimes, it seemed that they carried this to the extreme of avoiding topics which might have benefited from discussion.

Occasionally, there were indications of change having been consciously integrated into a reconstructed scale of values. One woman had advised a friend whose husband had meanwhile suffered an infarction. She said

> This friend I've told that you have to change your way of life and live a day at a time. Then you have to look round at the little things and take pleasure in them, instead of doing things in a hurry and looking forward to big things. You have to get things more in perspective She said I had helped her.

Many women in this series appeared to lack just this kind of support from friends. Consequently, they were all the more in need of support from professional services.

Views on Professional Services

Asking wives about husbands' communication with doctors and the feasibility of advice had revealed many doubts and reservations. At a later stage in the interviews a more conventional approach to assessing satisfaction with services was used, women being asked whether they considered that husbands had as much help from medical services and over return to work as they needed. Here, two thirds of wives expressed themselves as completely satisfied with help from medical services. Praise was almost invariably high for hospital inpatient services, although less so for follow-up arrangements by hospitals and general practitioners. Non-manual wives, despite their husbands' generally better outcome, were rather less often completely satisfied with medical services than were manual wives (Table 10.2).

One woman expressed much appreciation of the duplicated advice notes routinely given out by one ward. However she pointed out, that was on the occasion of her husband's second heart attack during the year. On the initial occasion he had been in another ward which gave no duplicated advice notes and, in retrospect, she now felt that this had been a great lack, possibly even contributing to the second attack. Another woman, who had no other criticisms, reported that her husband (a senior professional man) had found it very difficult to tie anyone in the ward down to advice on diet. Eventually a diet sheet had been produced but she felt that her husband should not have been made to appear to be fussing before he got it. A more frequent criticism was the lack of communication between hospital and general practitioners which caused uncertainty and engendered lack of confidence in the latter.

The level of satisfaction was lower over arrangements for return to work. Excluding those women whose husbands did not return to work, even temporarily, only one half of the remainder considered that husbands had received as much help as they needed, wives of non-manual workers in this case more often thinking arrangements adequate than did wives of manual workers (Table 10.3).

Despite criticisms, relatively few women had any definite ideas on how services could be changed for the better. One man had been in the process of changing jobs on medical advice just before infarction and lost, during his illness, the job he had been promised, subsequently finding for himself work which both he and his wife considered too tiring. His wife thought that 'the interviewers at the Labour Exchange should be better genned up because, if they don't know what is available, how can they tell someone at the other side of the counter . . . employment has been the biggest worry from beginning to end, both as the cause and continuing now'. As an incomer from a larger city, she was particularly critical of local services. Less articulate women with less experience of comparable services more often said, as they did also when referring to the limitations of their lay help and consultation systems, 'There is nothing anyone can do', with the implication that the main problems lay in husbands' personality and/or work situation, and that since these were perceived as unchangeable, further help from the services was not seen as relevant. This acceptance of what is seen as inevitable is in accordance with the findings of other studies such as that of Tizard, Rutter and Whitmore[6] where parents' expectations of help with their children's difficulties are low. In this connection Festinger[7] has pointed out that when people believe that they cannot change a situation, they often come to believe that they are satisfied with existing conditions, because it is only in this way that they can get rid of the sense of worry and unease arising from the wish to change something that they think is unchangeable.

These indications of needs unmet by community services twelve months after infarction are in sharp contrast with the confidence expressed in hospital services at the crisis. Deficiencies in communication provided a theme frequently recurring both in the relationship between spouses and in their contacts with services and with members of their informal social networks. Such deficiencies seemed to point to a need for professionals to take the initiative by anticipating the types of difficulty likely to arise and identifying families likely to be particularly at risk. Greater use of group therapy and counselling from early stages might reduce the need for more expensive forms of intervention later; rather than new services, better use of existing services seems necessary. This is discussed further in later chapters.

Notes

1. Mechanic, D. (1968). *Medical Sociology*, New York, Free Press.
2. Skelton, M. and Dominian, J. (1973). Psychological Stress in Wives of Patients with Myocardial Infarction. *British Medical Journal* 2, 101-3.
3. Thompson, B. and Finlayson, A. (1963). Married Women Who Work in Early Motherhood. *British Journal of Sociology* 14, 150-68.
4. Davis, M.S. (1969). Variations in Patients' Compliance with Doctors' Advice: An Empirical Analysis of Patterns of Communication. *American Journal of Public Health* 58, 274-88.
5. It may be apposite to say here that we were sometimes asked why we did not study recovery from heart disease in women. It is true that, although the incidence is much lower, especially before menopausal age, there are signs that it is increasing. Indeed, indications in this series point to an increase in heart ailments among wives during husbands' post-infarction career as well as increase in smoking and exposure to stress. However because the roles of men and women, both in work and family, are still so very different it would hardly have been possible to compare women's experience in respect of the contingencies on which we focused. A separate study of a series of women would, of course be useful — and perhaps not least if it were to reveal whether there exists any counterpart to the stereotype of the 'nagging wife' attributing causation perhaps to husbands, mothers, children, employers or others.
6. Tizard, J., Rutter, M. and Whitmore, K. (1970). *Education, Health and Behaviour*, London, Longman.
7. Festinger, L. (1962). *A Theory of Cognitive Dissonance*, London, Tavistock.

11 OUTCOME AT TWELVE MONTHS: OBJECTIVE AND SUBJECTIVE DEFINITIONS

So far, we have seen that many families faced considerable difficulties in the post-infarction career. Lemert,[1] using the career concept to refer to recurrent or typical contingencies awaiting patients, added the notion that there may be theoretically 'best' choices set into a situation by prevailing technology and social structure. In this series many families appeared at a disadvantage in respect of one or more contingencies and to lack opportunities to make 'best' choices. We can now ask whether any of the distinctions which we have drawn between families, either in terms of social characteristics present at infarction or in the way in which they coped with problems in the post-infarction career are related to outcome. If so, examination of such factors should make it easier to assess what kinds of men, in terms of their work, family and social situation, are most at risk of not achieving a successful outcome. This would open up for the future the possibility of initiating for such patients more positive and sustained follow-up procedures, perhaps using the goal-setting approach, which appears effective in rehabilitation after various other disabilities and especially in encouraging patients and professionals to work towards the same goals.

It may be appropriate to recapitulate here the definitions of outcome which we used at twelve months. In medical models, outcome has usually been taken as return or non-return to work. In pilot interviews it was clear that this had validity to the extent that women whose husbands were not back at work felt that outcome was largely defined by that fact. Women whose husbands were working, however, did not all accept that the illness was over. Accordingly, we have tried to combine objective and subjective criteria.

Twenty men in this series were not working twelve months later, that is just over one in every four. Just over half of these had been off work continuously while the others had returned but were off work again at the time of the second interview. Although it was still possible that some men would resume regular work their prospects of doing so appeared low in comparison with those who had been in continuous work and thus they could be considered on objective grounds as having had unsuccessful outcomes at this point. For the remaining three quarters we introduced a subjective criterion — the definition of a 'significant other', in this case the wife — as to whether the illness was over or not. In terms of this subjective criterion, wives of just over half these men thought that the illness was by and large, over or made very minor reservations, while the remainder considered that it was not over was 'still there' or 'still very much affecting him'. Thus we could distinguish three types of outcome: 'A', where men were back at work and wives considered the illness as over; 'B' where men were back at work but wives did not consider the illness as over; and 'C', where men were not back at work.

Social Class and Age

Considerable differences appeared between non-manual and manual families in respect of both objective and subjective criteria, both distinctions indicating a higher proportion of successful outcomes for non-manual families. Of the 28 non-manual men, over half had outcome 'A', one third 'B' and only four 'C' while, of the 48 manual workers, about one third fell into each category.

Outcome appeared also to be related to age in so far as the objective distinction between return to work and non-return ('A' and 'B as opposed to 'C') is concerned but less so in respect of the subjective distinction between 'A' and 'B' which show rather similar age distribution. Of the 13 men aged under 44, just under half were back at work compared with three quarters of those in the other age groups, among which those in the intermediate age group (45 - 54) achieved the highest rate, 88 per cent. This difference, however, is related to social class distribution since over the series as a whole a higher proportion of manual workers than of non-manual workers was aged under 44 (Tables 11.1 to 11.3).

Role Rearrangement and Outcome

In most respects the association between social class and outcome is closer than any association between characteristics or ways of coping with contingencies within either of the two social class groupings. This is not unexpected, since the type and conditions of work required seem more likely to be available in non-manual occupations while some of the adaptations required such as change in food habits may be less practicable for manual families. However there was one contingency in respect of which differences between the three outcome groups were sharper than that within social class groupings. This was the extent to which husbands' household tasks had been taken over (and were still being carried out at twelve months) by other family members. As is seen in Appendix 11.4, this occurred in three quarters of families in Social Classes I and II compared with just over half of manual families

Where men were not back at work — outcome 'C' — their household tasks appeared to have been taken over in only half the non-manual and under half the manual families (Table 11.4). Instead, some men who were fit enough and willing had taken on household tasks from their wives. In such instances of role reversal, wives were usually doing outside work (and had been doing this before infarction). Some women had been agreeably surprised at the readiness with which husbands had accepted such reversal and all felt that it increased the men's self-respect by giving them something useful to do. It also, of course made it easier for women to keep up outside work and more than one spoke, half seriously, of wondering how she would manage if her husband did, eventually, get back to work. Not all instances of role reversal, however, involved working wives. A number of other factors could also be operative. In the case of a baker, who was unable to return to hot and heavy night work and who had taken over all household cooking from his wife, his previous skill was clearly relevant. His wife's own uncertain health, the presence in the household of a school-age child, and the wages brought in by two adolescents were all contributory factors keeping her from seeking work. The fact that she was an incomer, who had moved to the area on marriage, may also have been relevant since a survey in a city of comparable size, Aberdeen, has shown that such women, lacking pre-marrriage experience of local jobs, are less likely to hear of work opportunities.[2]

Among families where husbands were back at work, wives who defined the illness as over (outcome 'A') also reported low rates for takeover of husbands' household tasks. Unlike the role reversal process in outcome group 'C', this was because many of these families had reached 'return-to-normality' and husbands had resumed household tasks as well as work roles. In sharp contrast, in families with outcome 'B', where husbands were at work but wives did not consider the illness as over, a very high proportion had taken on and had retained husbands' household tasks — every non-manual family in this group and three out of every four manual families.

These differences suggest that in families with outcome 'B' the wife's perception of the illness as not over is reflected in role changes which have the effect of releasing husbands from household tasks; in 'A' families the perception of the illness as being over means that there is less need for such change; and in families with outcome 'C', where husbands have not returned to work, changes have been more often in the direction of role reversal with some homebound husbands taking on tasks from their wives, who are generally, although not always, themselves working outside the home.

Where men had returned to work the differences between 'A' and B' families on takeover of husbands' house tasks seems also to correlate with wives' reports as to whether husbands had changed their working habits or conditions of employment. Among women who considered the illness as over, two out of every three of those married to non-manual workers reported change in work habits and a rather higher proportion of those married to manual workers. In contrast, where women did not perceive the illness as over, only one third of those married to non-manual workers and rather under one half of those married to manual workers reported sustained change in work habits. The implication would seem to be that women who perceived their husbands' illness as still operative and their work conditions as unchanged, tried to alter such conditions as lay within their power by freeing husbands from household tasks (Table 11.5).

Socio-Demographic Characteristics and Outcome

We also wanted to know whether any of the socio-demographic characteristics distinguishing between families at infarction appeared to be associated with outcome. In most respects differences related to class and age appeared more important than any other differences overall or within the two groupings. However, a number of factors which showed, in varying degrees, some association with outcome require examination. Among them, wives' work roles and wives' expectations showed some variations.

As was explained in Chapter 10, wives' work roles were not greatly altered in the course of the post-infarction career. It might never the less be suggested that since, overall, full-time working wives were less frequently married to men who had returned to work (just over half compared with four in every five among part-time working wives and even more among full-time housewives) then full-time work by wives might constitute an adverse factor contributing to poor outcome. This association can, however, be partially explained by the fact that manual workers more often than non-manual men, had working wives and partially by age differences within each of the social class groupings. Among non-manual families the age factor was important, all four of the men not back at work being aged over 55 and thus rather readier to think of retirement; three of their wives were, already before the illness, working full-time and the other part-time. One of the full-time workers who was several years younger than her husband, explained that, when he had been seriously ill with artery trouble some years previously, she had decided to work full-time and that he encouraged this because he felt that her future would be more secure if anything happened to him (Table 11.6).

Among the wives of manual workers, the proportion of full-time housewives remained around one in four for all types of outcome and there was little difference in the proportion of full-time working wives for outcomes 'A' and 'C' (although there was a high proportion of part-time workers for outcome 'B'). Here the more interesting finding is the clustering of wives who normally worked full-time but who were either out of work or unfit for work at one or both interviews. Of the eight women not working at second interview who normally went out to work, six were married to men who were themselves not back at work — outcome 'C' — and the other two husbands were in the intermediate category outcome 'B'. Six of the eight women (not always the same ones) had been off work at the time of their husbands' infarction. Thus, unfavourable outcome for manual workers seemed to be associated rather with poor socio-economic conditions in which wives were unemployed or unfit for work than with the fact that wives normally worked.

Wives' expectations also presented a somewhat complex picture. At the time of husbands' hospitalisation women had been asked about their expectations in relation to particular contingencies and they were not asked whether they expected the illness to be over at any particular time. (This was to obviate any suggestion that there was some kind of norm when the illness might be expected to be over.) Wives who had anticipated no difficulties in respect of any of the denoted contingencies (work, leisure, smoking, money and consulting doctor) had been considered to have very favourable expectations while those anticipating difficulties in respect of all, or all but one contingency, were considered as having very unfavourable expectations. One can ask, therefore, whether outcome varied with these expectations (Table 11.7).

Among non-manual families where one half of the wives reported favourable expectations on four or five contingencies this did appear to be the case, eight of their husbands achieving outcome 'A', four 'B' and only two 'C' (both the latter being older men close to retiring age). Among the considerably smaller proportion of manual wives who expressed four or five favourable expectations, less than one quarter, there is no such trend, only two of the ten husbands having outcome 'A', five 'B' and three 'C'.

If, however, one looks at wives who were very pessimistic (expressing favourable expectations on only one contingency, or on no contingencies at all), then of the fourteen manual wives who did so, only two were married to men who subsequently achieved outcome 'A', compared with five and seven having outcomes 'B' and 'C' respectively. (Only one non-manual wife had expectations as low as this group and her husband had outcome 'B'.) Thus it seemed that overall the social class dichotomy was more important than wives' expectations in predicting outcome, but, among non-manual families, favourable expectations by wives were associated with successful outcome and, among manual families, exceptionally unfavourable expectations were associated with unsuccessful outcome. That is, wives' expectations could help to pick out the extremes at either end but were not, by themselves, effective in the middle ranges.

Looking back on first interviews, one could see that some optimistic wives had been unrealistic in overestimating the degree of change and adaptation that they were expecting both of their husbands and of work situations, while others, more cautious at first interview, had been pleasantly surprised by finding resources in their husbands or in their work or family situations which they had not recognised at the time of crisis. Wives' expectations had, however, also been taken into account as part of the investigator's assessment of 'areas of potential stress' and this provided a better association with outcome as shown below.

Outcome Related to Areas of Potential Stress

As noted in Chapter 5 it seemed to us that many men appeared to be starting out on their post-infarction careers already handicapped by carrying with them an excessive burden of on-going problems even although they and their wives did not always make these explicit. We were in agreement with the view of Rosenstock[3] that illness behaviour takes place in a context where motives are frequently competing or in conflict, and had noted Querido's[4] finding of a significant difference between hospital patients who had to cope with problems apart from their physical illness and those who did not.

For these reasons, assessment was made after first interviews as to whether each family showed evidence of potential stress in any of five different areas and whether these conditions seemed likely to continue into the post-infarction career. These areas were: (1) the existence of intercurrent serious illness of the husband other than the infarction itself; (2) difficulties likely to arise for the husband at work or in return to work; (3) difficulties relating to the husband's personality or the wife's perception of it; (4) difficulties in the nuclear family, e.g. health problems of wife or child, adolescent troubles of more than average seriousness; (5) difficulties in the social network surrounding the family, e.g. elderly kin who presented health problems or who made excessive demands, or active disagreement with neighbours.

On this basis, half the non-manual families and two thirds of the manual families were assessed as being exposed to three or more 'areas of potential stress'. When these families were later compared with those for whom only two or fewer areas were scored there appeared to be an association between number of areas scored and outcome. Families having outcome 'A' had scored fewest areas of stress the number increasing through 'B' to 'C' and this holds, as shown in Table 11.8, for both non-manual and manual families, while, within each category, manual families had scored more areas of stress than non-manual families. Furthermore, if we consider families for whom four or five areas are scored then there is a very steep gradient for manual families.

Apart from these overall scores indicating a generally high level of potential stress, families could also be compared in respect of individual areas of stress. Then, as shown in Table 11.9, work difficulties and network difficulties produce gradients in which high scores increase with poor outcome, the former within social class and the latter overall; nuclear family difficulties produce a gradient increasing with poor outcome for manual families and a high level in 'B' non-manual families; husbands' pre-infarction illness is concentrated for non-manual men in outcomes 'B' and 'C' and for manual workers in 'C'. Only husbands' personality difficulties, having a very high overall rate, show little overall difference with outcome, not indeed with class.

Thus it seemed that assessment of areas of potential stress at the time of hospitalisation, coupled with information on age and socio-economic status, could help to indicate men likely to have less successful outcomes. Such assessment could be undertaken by medical social workers or by health visitors who would then be in a position to collaborate with general practitioners in initiating and sustaining programmes of intervention.

Ordinal Position and Outcome

A more unexpected finding emerging from analysis of this series is an apparent effect of ordinal position in manual families and it is tentatively suggested that it might be worth looking at this factor in larger studies. It has already been mentioned in Chapter 5 that the family size of both husbands and wives over the series as a whole appeared rather high and that this was more so in respect of men, with their relative shortage of family sizes one and two and relative excess of sizes five to seven than in respect of their wives. Thus, because large family size is known to be associated with physical and social disadvantage, we thought that it might also predispose to poor outcome. This did not, however prove to be the case, except in so far as large family size was related to manual work status.

Ordinal position, however, both in representation in the series and in outcome, showed some anomalies and, although numbers are recognised to be small, it seems worth drawing attention to them (Tables 11.10 and 11.11). The first is that there appears to be an underrepresentation of men who were eldest children, since irrespective of the number of intermediate and only children, the number of eldests and youngests in a series should be approximately equal. In this series this is true (or more true) of wives (who can again serve as controls), there being 18 eldests and 21 youngests among the wives of the 76 men survivors (or, if men who died during the year are included bringing the total to 88, then 22 wives are eldests and 23 are youngests). The men's pattern contrasts with this for only 15 out of 76 survivors are eldests while 21 are youngests (more strikingly, if men dying during the year are included to bring the total to 88 there are still only 15 eldests while the number of youngests increases to 25). Does this suggest that it might be worth looking at ordinal position in studies of myocardial infarction with larger populations to see whether eldests more often die at a very early stage in the illness and are thus underrepresented in a population of survivors like this one or, alternatively, whether men who are eldests less often suffer myocardial infarction?

The second anomaly is the rather curious distribution in relation to outcome of such eldests as do appear in this series. Seven of the eldests among the survivors were manual workers who experienced outcome 'C', where they constituted 44 per cent of that outcome.

It has been suggested that, in manual families eldest males may be socially disadvantaged in having to take on instrumental roles and to become responsible parent substitutes and wage-earners at an earlier age than other family members. It may be that the kind of work into which they are pushed for immediate financial advantage may be just that to which it is difficult to return after serious illness. An interesting comparison is afforded by the fact that, of the eighteen women who are eldests, seven are concentrated in manual 'A' families where they form half of that outcome. Does this suggest that, in contrast to the instrumental role allotted to the male who is eldest in manual families, the female who is the eldest in a manual family is socialised into a nurturing, expressive role which later is adapted to promote the wellbeing of her husband. Women married to eldests and women who were themselves eldests often appeared to see this family position as involving responsibilities rather than privileges and some sense of eldests being exploited by parents was not far below the surface.

Clausen[5] who has summarised many studies of ordinal position, has reported that the effects are still not understood. He found, however, in his own study evidence that eldest children had more often received physical punishment than other children, especially if they were in large families. Tizard, Rutter and Whitmore found that children in their study showing neurotic symptoms were more often eldests and less often youngests.[6] A number of studies have shown that parents report themselves more relaxed with later children. Earlier studies have found eldests to be more often successful in educational and occupational terms than others. It may be that most previous studies have been deficient in failing to distinguish between possible differences in the meaning of ordinal position in manual as opposed to non-manual families.

Congruence of Definitions and Outcome

In this chapter we have shown that differences in outcome at twelve months, whether this is defined objectively as return-to-work or subjectively to include perception of the illness as being over or not, were associated with changed behaviour patterns in families in respect of household tasks formerly carried out by husbands. We have also suggested that differences in outcome, again defined in both ways, appeared to be associated with some factors distinguishing between families which were noted at the beginning of the post-infarction career, particularly social class, age and the extent of areas of potential stress. These three factors serve to pick out families where difficulties appear particularly acute.

A further factor appearing to discriminate against a substantial number of families has been touched on earlier. This is the extent to which definitions made early in the post-infarction career by members of the social networks surrounding the family appeared to be congruent with professional definitions. Some illustrations of how this process works were given in Chapter 6 but such material does not lend itself directly to quantitative analysis. However, one way of classifying networks in terms of women's lay help and consultation patterns has been attempted and is described in the following chapter. It points to an association between poor outcomes and restricted networks where congruence with professional definitions appeared less likely and where relatively ineffective support appeared available for coping with difficulties and problems encountered in the post-infarction career.

Notes

1. Lemert, E.M. (1967). *Human Deviance, Social Problems & Social Control,* Englewood Cliffs, New Jersey, Prentice Hall Inc.
2. Thompson, B. and Finlayson, A. (1963). Married Women Who Work in Early Motherhood. *British Journal of Sociology* 14, 150-68.
3. Rosenstock, I.M. *et al.* (1959). Why People Fail to Seek Poliomyelitis Vaccination. *Public Health Reports* 74, 98-103.
4. Querido, A. (1959). An Investigation into the Clinical, Social, and Mental Factors Determining the Results of Hospital Treatment. *British Journal of Social and Preventive Medicine* 13, 33-49.
5. Clausen, J. (1966). Family Structure, Socialisation & Personality. In Hofmann, M.L. & L.W. (ed.). *Review of Child Development Research,* Russell Sage Foundation.
6. Tizard, J., Rutter, M. and Whitmore, K. (1970). *Education, Health and Behaviour,* London, Longman.

12 SOCIAL NETWORKS AS COPING RESOURCES: WIVES' HELPERS AND LAY CONSULTANTS

We considered the use of social networks as coping resources to be a main focus for the study, the more so since experience in teaching students of medicine, nursing, social administration and applied social studies had made us aware of the difficulties in interpreting the concept of social network in a way that appears relevant to present and future workers in health and social services. Although lip-service is increasingly paid to the importance of 'the family' and 'significant others' in supporting the individual, there have been so far few attempts to study in a systematic way the contribution made by different categories of family members and friends in times of crisis or long-term difficulties. Small wonder then that, even when doctors are aware of the importance of social factors, they often consider it sufficient to warn students to recognise the role of 'granny' or 'the neighbours' in undermining (less often reinforcing) medical regimens and professional definitions; seldom going further to suggest that, in any given family, it may also be important to discover whether, for instance, 'granny' is mother's mother or father's mother and whether neighbours are seen as helpful or the reverse. The voluminous literature of sociology and social work emphasises the support afforded by a warm, close-knit network and has brought out particularly the strength of the tie between mothers and daughters. Relatively little attention has been devoted to other relationships in social networks and the kinds of support which professional workers might expect them to provide.

Two studies which we had tried to use as teaching material suggested useful insights but seemed limited in their application. The distinction drawn by Bott[1] between families with joint roles and loose-knit networks on one hand and those with segregated roles and close-knit networks on the other is quoted in many textbooks both of sociology and social work; in her second edition[2] Bott, referring to the many families which appear to be intermediate between the two extremes, suggests that attempts should be made to classify families according to the amount of help which women receive in a family crisis and according to the persons who act as helpers. McKinlay[3] has used the concept of social network as a lay referral system to explain his findings that, among pregnant women married to unskilled workers, those with close-knit networks and those who consult relatives over problems are less likely to make good use of medical services than are those women who consult husbands or other persons.

We thought that it would be valuable to identify in the context of a crisis those persons who were perceived by women as giving immediate practical help and also those whom they anticipated using as consultants in any future problems. We were interested particularly in the extent to which persons perceived as helpers overlapped with those seen as consultants and the way in which patterns might change over twelve months. In addition, this series of families, differing from those studied by Bott and McKinlay in being at a later stage in the family life cycle, offered a useful opportunity for beginning to examine the role of adult children. Our interest in the latter had been aroused while carrying out an earlier survey into a difficult aspect of occupational health, which depended upon obtaining the co-operation of respondents in older age groups.[4] In the course of that survey, we had noted that the influence of the younger generation was sometimes evident in encouraging respondents to co-operate even when that of respondents' siblings might be discouraging ('my sister said I shouldna see you but my son said I should'); the younger generation seemed to be making assumptions about the purpose of the survey and its usefulness which were more congruent with professional definitions. We wondered whether, in the context of an ongoing crisis, similar differences in attitudes between younger and older family members might emerge and whether they might affect compliance with medical regimens.

During first interviews, wives were asked to name persons who were of help to them while their husbands were in hospital; a year later they were asked who had been of help during the year following their husbands' return from hospital; at the time of hospitalisation they were also asked with whom they expected to talk over difficulties if any should arise during husbands' recovery; a year later they were asked with whom they currently discussed any problems or difficulties.

Differences in the availability of kin were indicated in Chapter 5. Recognition of the importance of this structural factor enabled us to discuss with women some reasons for their choices; for instance the process of substitution described by Townsend[5] could be seen to be operating where a sister or mother-in-law had taken over a role earlier played by a deceased mother.

Although the identification of specific individuals was valuable for qualitative assessment of networks and has been used as an illustration in other chapters, our emphasis, for quantitative analysis in this chapter, was placed on the representation or absence of each category as a source of support or help, regardless of the number of persons named or the positions named, within that category. This was done for two reasons; first, to simplify analysis, and, second, because we considered that members of an individual's family of origin, having shared a common socialisation process, were likely also to share a consensus of expectations about that individual, e.g. 'Tom is such a worrier', 'Bill is so sensible', 'Jack will never stop smoking' — the effect of which was likely to be cumulative. We expected that variations between mother and sister would be minor compared with the variation between any member of that category and a member of other categories.

Persons named as helpers and consultants were considered as representing the following categories (or sources) of support or help: children (including sons-in-law and daughters-in-law); members of wife's family of origin (wife's kin); members of husbands' family of origin (husband's kin); and 'others', i.e. non-kin. As consultants, husbands could also be named.

We did not think that it would be realistic to restrict women to selecting one principal consultant only. They were, therefore, able to choose persons from more than one category. Consequently, it was not possible to separate the women themselves as McKinlay had done, into mutually exclusive types, some choosing husbands only and others choosing mothers or sisters only. We were, however, able to make comparisons between groups of women in terms of the extent to which individual categories were represented, as well as in the number of categories represented, thus showing differences in the total range of network members who played the roles of helper or consultant and also suggesting why some families lacked such members and others did not use them.

The details, which are complex, are shown in Tables 12.1 to 12.6. It is recognised that when a small series is broken down by a combination of variables, the use of percentages becomes hazardous. This particularly applied to the non-manual 'C' group which includes only 4 families. However if this group were to be combined with non-manual 'B', the differences would still be in the required direction.

Lay Help Patterns

Nearly all women reported receiving some help during the time that husbands were in hospital and some were almost overwhelmed by offers of assistance. The kind of help needed varied according to individual circumstances, including, for instance, driving wives to hospital, baby-sitting, having children to stay, preparing meals, telephoning or providing access to a telephone, reassuring husbands or wives about employment prospects, inviting wives who were nervous about being alone at night to stay or coming to stay with them, and just 'being there' (Table 12.1).

Overall, one third of the women reported help from one source (or category) only; a slightly larger number acknowledged persons from two different categories and one quarter referred to persons from three or four different categories. Access to this wide range of three or four categories was more often claimed by non-manual wives (over one third reporting this) than by wives of manual workers (one in every five reporting this). (As indicated earlier, each category might comprise more than one person so the total number of individuals giving help was, of course, much greater.)

When the number of sources of help at the crisis was later related to outcome, it was found that over one third of families with outcome 'A' had reported help from three or more sources compared with one quarter of 'B' families and only one in ten of 'C' families ('A' families being those where husbands were back at work a year later and where wives defined the illness as over; 'B' families being those where wives did not consider the illness as over although husbands were back at work; and 'C' families where husbands were not back at work). If in addition, different types of outcome are combined with differences between classes, then, as shown in Table 12.1, help from three or more sources at the crisis was reported by nearly half of all non-manual 'A' women but, at the other extreme, by only one woman out of sixteen manual families with outcome 'C'.

A year later, when wives were asked who had been of help to them during the year since husbands' return from hospital, the number of sources mentioned had declined considerably, as would be expected, less than one third now naming two or more sources of help and ten women naming no one (Table 12.2). Some said that they had needed no help while others, although clearly still worried, put it that 'there is nothing that anyone can do'.

Thus, right from the beginning, manual families could be seen as having access to a narrower range of informal support; and, after twelve months, a sharp contrast had emerged between the two extremes in this respect — those non-manual families who had the most favourable outcomes having had access from early days to the greatest range of informal help while those manual families who had least favourable outcomes had been more restricted in the range of informal help available to them.

Analysis of the frequency with which different categories of help were mentioned at first interview showed that, overall, nearly half the women named helpers from their own kin, usually mothers or sisters one third mentioned husband's kin, three out of every five named children and the same percentage named 'others' (Table 12.3).

In the light of many studies on the relationship between kinship and class (summarised in Bott[1]), we expected that there would be differences between manual and non-manual families in the frequency with which different categories would be named. This can be clearly seen in respect of 'others', i.e. non-kin, these being named much more often by non-manual than manual women. The type of help which was forthcoming from this category also varied. When manual women did mention 'others' these were generally neighbours or workmates proffering immediate help, such as use of car or telephone or the provision of child-care or meals, types of assistance which were essentially of a short-term character. Non-manual wives, in contrast, more often mentioned, in addition to friends and acquaintances who encouraged them with accounts of successful recoveries, considerable support from husbands' work associates — employers, managers partners — who reassured the family about the work situation in a way that had long-term implications.

In respect of the other categories, however, variations between classes, as such, appeared small. Instead, the overall picture concealed variations which related to differences later found in the outcome of the illness. As Table 12.3 shows just over two thirds of the families who later had outcome 'A' reported help from children. The reasons for a corresponding deficiency among 'C' families (where only one in four of the non-manual and fewer than half the manual wives mentioned children) seem to be, at least in part, structural, two of these couples being childless, two having handicapped adult children only, while other families had children who were either too young to help or, alternatively, children who had migrated from the district. Furthermore, families with outcome 'C' appeared to be deficient in at least one other source of help — non-manual families in respect of wife's kin and manual 'C' families in respect of husband's kin. Again, the reasons appeared to be largely structural, age factors and migration playing a part in this.

At second interviews, twelve months later, it was noticeable that, although help from children had remained at almost the same level overall, assistance from wives' kin had fallen markedly (Table 12.4). This decline was particularly pronounced for manual families with outcome 'C' and, although the latter recorded slightly increased help from children, this was by no means sufficient to compensate, being still appreciably lower than that recorded for those manual families who had outcomes 'A' and 'B'. There seemed some evidence that, even where no structural deficiencies caused by death or migration existed, kin and children in this group might more often play a dependent or negative role rather than a supportive one, e.g. 'My sister more often comes to me for help' or 'My mother's too old now'.

Among non-manual wives, two, both with outcome 'A', who worked in partnership with self-employed husbands and who had employees and prosperous customers, seemed aware of receiving more support than two wives who shared with their husbands businesses which were marginally viable; one of these latter families had outcome 'B' and one 'C'. Another two wives, whose networks had been outstandingly supportive, were both married to senior professional men whose work and interests had clearly involved them in many reciprocal ties in their communities. Some of the non-manual wives with husbands in commercial or industrial occupations received markedly less support, and sometimes there were indications that husband's colleagues were little known or were seen as competitors; however, one firm was described as being 'sentimental to all its employees' and another was said to have reorganised work under a new manager because 'too many heart attacks and illnesses among employees' had been occurring during the previous manager's tenure of office.

Lay Consultation Patterns

In general, it seemed that wives, while ready to accept offers of help from a variety of sources, when they took on the active role of confiding in or consulting someone, selected from a more limited field. To some extent, they appeared to be making a distinction between the many who approached them volunteering to fulfil an immediate, instrumental role and the few whom they themselves sought out to fulfil a more long-term, expressive role.

Comparison with the lay help pattern was complicated by the

fact that, since the husband's illness was the cause of the crisis, husbands could not be named as helpers at that time, although a few were mentioned as such a year later, generally when wives themselves had meanwhile been ill. Husbands were, however, often named both as anticipated and actual consultant, thus adding a fifth category.

At first interview, women were asked with whom they expected to talk over difficulties if any should arise in the course of husband's recovery. Overall, members of their own kin (nearly always a mother or sister) were selected by approximately two out of every five women; one third chose husbands and a slightly smaller number chose 'others' (rather less than half the latter naming professional persons). Children and husbands' kin were mentioned relatively seldom and four women could think of no one whom they would consult. (Percentages in Table 12.5 add up to more than 100 because, as with helpers, some women mentioned consultants from two or three different categories.)

Again, as one would expect from previous studies (summarised in Bott) the main differences were associated with social class, non-manual wives more often mentioning husbands and manual wives more often mentioning their own kin.

Among the 'others' named were several professional persons. These included general practitioners and a few nurses (the latter all holding the dual role of neighbour), as well as one minister of religion and one priest. Non-professional 'others' included neighbours, workmates and friends other than those already included as neighbours and workmates.

At second interview the question was not restricted to husbands' illness (because some women might feel that this raised no difficulties requiring discussion). Instead, women were asked with whom they usually, currently, talked over any problems or worries. This time, as Table 12.6 shows, there was an increase of 10 per cent in the number mentioning husbands which might be because, at first interview, some wives had been anticipating the need for discussing his illness with some one other than himself and had now reverted to a pre-infarction pattern.

At the same time, the percentage naming a member of their own kin had fallen from two in every five to one quarter, children were mentioned by one in every five, husband's kin by 11 per cent and 'others' by 16 per cent. Eighteen women, that is nearly one in every four, said that they consulted no one, either having no 'real' problems or keeping them to themselves; this was a very sharp increase on the four women who had named no one at first interview and is discussed further below in relation to class and outcome.

Non-manual wives again mentioned husbands much more often than any other category, while manual wives named their own kin slightly more often than either husbands or children. In the diminished category of 'others' no women now claimed to consult professional persons and, among manual wives, only four now mentioned 'others' at all. Altogether, the earlier expectations of many women appeared to have been unrealistic.

Lay Consultation in Relation to Outcome

Looking at the consultation patterns in relation to outcome then, as shown in Table 12.6, the characteristic within non-manual families which appeared to differentiate 'A' families from 'B' and 'C' was the greater consulting of husbands.

Among manual families, the characteristic that appeared to differentiate 'A' families was the greater consulting of children. Moreover, this had increased from first interview, whereas in manual 'B' families the rate was the same as at first interview and children were only named by one manual 'C' wife compared with two at first interview. This suggests that some manual wives with outcome 'A', who had thought of their children as sources of help but not as possible consultants at the crisis, had since found them capable of the additional role. It also suggests that, particularly in manual families, if such children are perceived as having acquired some wider experience outside the family — perhaps because of improved or extended education and/or upward mobility — they may be influential in changing expectations and behaviour in parents hitherto confined to closeknit networks and less flexible role expectations.

At the other extreme, among manual families with outcome 'C' there is some evidence of unrealistic expectations at first interview, particularly in relation to wife's family of origin, three out of every five women mentioning a mother or sister at the time while, at second interview, fewer than two out of every five named them. Sometimes a mother was seen as being now 'too old to burden her with my troubles', or a sister as having 'enough problems with her own family', these being perceptions which emerge as the result of a long drawn out experience of misfortune but which may not be apparent at the time of crisis.

The distribution of the eighteen women (nearly one in four, overall) who said at second interview that they consulted no one further points up the contrast between the two extremes. This was

said by only one non-manual wife out of the fifteen whose husbands
had outcome 'A' (7 per cent), compared with seven manual wives out
of the sixteen whose husbands had outcome 'C' (44 per cent). Women
married to manual workers who had outcome 'A' had the next
lowest percentage (14 per cent) and percentages among women married
to men experiencing the other three outcomes clustered between
22 per cent and 28 per cent.

A few of these women, especially one or two whose husbands'
work had kept them away from home a good deal, prided themselves
on being, by nature and habit, more independent than most people
and thus less in need of consultants. More often, however, women,
although perhaps not entirely isolated in the sense that nearly all
acknowledged accepting offers of practical help, expressed regret at
having no one to act as consultant. Some women spoke of missing
their mothers, even if these had died several years previously. One
woman illustrated the difficulties felt by those who may have
previously been very dependent and who have little experience in
forming new relationships and articulating needs:

I don't like to ask any one for help — if my mum had been alive
I wouldn't have had to ask her — she'd have been here. . .I keep
things to myself. . .My sister looked after my husband when he
was better for a week, while I went to stay with my daughter
after her baby was born, but I don't tell them things because I
think everyone has enough of their own troubles.

Other women explained that their mothers were now too old or
unwell, that they had enough troubles of their own(one looked after
her mother aged ninety) or that they lived too far away. One woman,
an incomer from England, said that her mother-in-law, who had
been the person she confided in when her husband was first ill, was
now herself seriously ill, which of course, added to her own and her
husband's worries.

Occasionally, women admitted that they were not on good terms
with their mothers and this was also sometimes said about sisters,
one or two being described as 'more my mother's favourite'. Other
women said that their sisters had enough to do looking after their
own families and, in a few instances, sisters were responsible for
elderly fathers, thus sparing respondents of this care. One woman
spoke of the effect of a handicapped child as having made herself
and her husband very independent of other people, so that, although

they themselves gave considerable help to elderly relatives, they did not confide in them.

Disadvantages of Networks Restricted to Families of Origin

This is a small series and generalisations from it should not be pushed too far. However, it seems that wives whose husbands had successful outcomes (husbands at work and wives defining illness as over) tended to be those who acknowledged support (in terms of lay help and consultation) from a wider range of sources, among whom husbands and non-kin appeared important for non-manual families and adult children appeared important for manual families. Conversely, wives whose husbands had less successful outcomes tended to be those who acknowledged support from a narrower range of sources, often restricted to kin of one or both spouses.

Other factors, reported in earlier chapters, also appeared relevant and it is not suggested that there is a causal connection between lay help and consultation patterns and outcome. Nevertheless, to a large extent, these findings are in the same direction as those of McKinlay who showed that, among pregnant wives of unskilled workers those who consulted husbands or non-kin over problems were more often utilisers of services than were those who consulted relatives, and may thus suggest that the types of lay referral systems which are conducive to utilisation may also be conducive to successful outcome.

However, in this series where most families were at a later stage in the family life cycle than were those studied by McKinlay, the role of adult children as a source of sustained help or, more unusually, as lay consultants has been shown to be particularly important for manual families.

This suggests the possibility that, for manual families, the presence in the lay referral system of adult children, who have been exposed to longer education and more diversified influences, may increase congruence with professional definitions and encourage utilisation of services and adherence to professional advice, as well as facilitating change of expectations and roles within the family. In contrast, the absence in manual families of adult children (or their not being perceived as supportive) often effectively limits the lay referral system to members of the families of origin of one or both spouses; such persons will be older and likely to be more limited in their social experience, tending to reinforce each others' resistance to professional definitions, to discourage or delay utilisation of services and also to retain rigid expectations about roles in the family.

We think that professional workers needing to estimate the informal support available to families may find it useful systematically to check the presence, or absence, of perceived support from each of the five sources, or categories, used in this study: adult children; wife's kin; husband's kin; non-kin; and spouse. This may indicate something of the total range and type of support, revealing deficiences requiring compensatory intervention. As we suggest in Chapter 15, such intervention need not necessarily prove unduly demanding on professional resources if expatients with favourable outcomes and their families and friends could be brought in as new network members.

This way of trying to quantify one aspect of social networks has been exploratory rather than within the main stream of sociological research on the family. Attempts at quantification sometimes can appear rather remote from 'the real world'. The differences shown to exist in this chapter do, however, appear to reflect something of the differing quality of informal support surrounding individual families which is implicit in the wives' accounts quoted here and in earlier chapters. It may be that a similar approach could prove useful both in research and in application to rehabilitation programmes where persons are adapting to varying types of disability or where they are chronically sick or elderly. Although this study was made in the context of a medical problem the approach may also have some applicability to the more general issue of the role of network members in fostering or hindering the acceptance of innovation and may thus have implications for social policy and social work as well as for medical practice.

Notes

1. Bott, E. (1957). *Family and Social Network: Roles, Norms and External Relationships in Ordinary Urban Families.* 1st edn., London, Tavistock.
2. Bott, E. (1971). *Family and Social Network*, ibid., 2nd edn. London, Tavistock.
3. McKinlay, J. (1973). Social Networks and Utilization Behaviour, *Social Forces,* 51 275-92.
4. Finlayson, A., McEwen, J. and Mair, A. (1971). Home Interviews with Relatives of Deceased Persons: A Means of Obtaining Histories of Exposure to a Hazardous Substance. *Scottish Medical Journal* 16, 509-12.
5. Townsend, P. (1963). *The Family Life of Old People,* Harmondsworth, Penguin.

13 LONG-TERM PERSPECTIVE : FOUR-YEAR FOLLOW-UP

Interviews with men and their wives during the year following myocardial infarction indicated that assessment of the impact of the illness could only be incomplete at twelve months since substantial processes of change and adaptation still appeared to be taking place. Accordingly, four years after infarction, records were checked and the survivors still living in the area were interviewed (Table 13.1). This final interview afforded an opportunity to see the post-infarction career in a long-term perspective. Relatively few studies in this field have been able to follow up patients over this period of time. (For administrative reasons it was not possible to make provision for a parallel programme of interviews with wives at this time. Changes in family expectations and roles, as perceived by the men, were, however, among the areas covered and, in some instances, wives were present during interviews.)

Of the eighty-eight men who had constituted the original study population, 67 per cent were alive and were interviewed. A further 9 per cent living outside the area were not interviewed. Deaths from heart disease accounted for 22 per cent and one man had died of other causes. Altogether three quarters of those who suffered a first myocardial infarction were alive four years later (compared with 86 per cent who were alive at twelve months). As this study commenced with a selected population, i.e. those discharged from hospital, and since the numbers are small, the survival rates must be interpreted with caution. There are only minor variations in survival in the different age groups below fifty-five years of age, but after that there appears to be a real increase in mortality, with only 52 per cent in the age group 55-60 being alive at four years.

Quality of Life

More relevant to this study, however, is the quality of life for the survivors. Long-term aspects of this are considered below in relation to the fifty-nine survivors living in or near Dundee and available for interview at four years.

An important finding was the considerable number of men who still complained of symptoms which they considered were related to their illness (Table 13.2). Two out of every three men complained of pain in the chest, most of them referring to it as angina (no attempt was made to check on the exact nature of the pain). Over one third complained of additional symptoms such as breathlessness and tiredness which they associated with their heart disease. Overall, one in ten regarded their symptoms as severe and very limiting, some of the remainder as mildly limiting.

During the four years, over one quarter had experienced further distinct episodes of illness attributed to their heart condition which had required medical care, and for nearly one in five men this had necessitated hospital readmission (Table 13.3). A slightly greater number, over one third, had experienced episodes of other illness (minor illness, such as colds, 'flu, diarrhoea, etc., were excluded) with rather fewer than one in five men requiring hospital admission.

Just as there was evidence of some recurring illness and continuing symptomatology, there were also reports of continuing medical treatment (Table 13.4). At the time of interview half the men said that they were still receiving treatment for their heart condition, but only about one in seven was currently being treated for other conditions.

This pattern of continued illness and symptoms had rather less effect on the employment record than might perhaps have been expected (Table 13.5). Three out of every four said that they had lost no time off work attributable to heart conditions during the period since they had returned to work following their myocardial infarction. During the same period two thirds had lost no time attributable to other conditions (minor illnesses generating one or two days absence again being excluded).

While these reports do not amount to an overall description of serious incapacitating illness, the continuance of symptoms and treatment in a considerable number of men shows that there has been not so much a 'return to normality' as a gradual acceptance of the presence of symptoms and the regular ingestion of tablets as part of a new 'normal' pattern of life.

Work Roles

At first glance, the work situation appeared much more satisfactory, nine out of ten being at work while only 2 per cent were unemployed and only 8 per cent unable to work at the time of interview because of sickness (Table 13.6). None of the men interviewed had retired prematurely. It is known, however, that among those who had left the

district and were thus not available for interview there were a few
early retirements.

Of the six men who at the time of interview were not working,
three had not worked at all since infarction and three had worked for
some time. One of the latter had also completed a year's course of
clerical retraining and had been undergoing further retraining, when
he suffered his third infarction shortly before interview. (It should be
noted that, although some of the men who were not working at
twelve months had subsequently returned to work, four of the nine
men who died between twelve months and four years had not been
working at twelve months and had almost certainly never returned.)

As indicated earlier, we consider return to work, in itself, to be
an insufficiently sensitive criterion which requires to be qualified by
more detailed examination of the working situation and the degree
of change entailed (Table 13.7). Of those working at four years,
nearly three out of every five were in the same employment as before
infarction; a further one in five were still in the employment to which
they had moved following infarction but which differed from their
previous employment. One quarter had experienced one or more
changes of employment during the post-infarction career. (Again,
it should be remembered that we are here looking at a population of
survivors. If we revert momentarily to another way of considering
the figures, the full effect of myocardial infarction can be seen
when it is realised that, out of the total original series of eighty-eight
men discharged from hospital, only one third survived in their former
employment four years later.)

Occupational mobility has been the result of a number of factors,
sometimes several combining to produce the final change. Decisions
by employers were involved in three out of every four changes;
decisions by the men themselves in under one half; and the medical
advice in under one quarter. In this respect, there is marked contrast
with reports at infarction, especially at six months, when optimistic
definitions had been made. Some men who had been aware, in the
months before infarction, of redundancy as being in varying degrees
at least a possibility, spoke at six months of this threat as having
receded, seemingly reassured that their employers would feel obliged
to retain them. In the event, their earlier pessimistic, definitions
proved the more realistic.

Although there was evidence that some of this occupational change
had been seen as stressful at earlier stages, the results at four years
appeared very satisfactory. All of those working said that they were

managing their work, nearly all reported that they were personally satisfied with their jobs and only one quarter said that they had any difficulties — in most cases, these not being severe. This satisfactory position appears to have been brought about by a fundamental process of adaptation, two out of every five reporting that they had reduced their average hours of work, usually as a result of undertaking less overtime (Table 13.8). Many, as we see later, had received a great deal of help and support initially from both management and fellow workers in their working situation and were still accorded practical help when and if it was required.

Self-help and help from informal resources were important in the negotiation of occupational change. Of those who were required to find a new job over half had obtained it themselves. Over one quarter had found work through the help or advice of friends and fewer than one in five through the Department of Employment. In general, relatively little use had been made of any of the official services, one quarter having had some contact with the Disablement Resettlement Officer, one in ten attending some form of rehabilitation course and only one in twenty having been in contact with social services. The few men who contacted occupational health services commented on the value of reassurance and of receiving practical help and advice in the work setting.

Leisure and Family Roles

Although new work roles and new satisfaction in work after initial difficulties had been achieved by most men this kind of positive adaptation did not generally extend to leisure and family roles. Men in this series reported a dramatic reduction in social and physical activity following infarction and this was still very evident at four years (physical activity performed at work is excluded here (Table 13.9)). One in every two men undertook fewer activities, went out less often, had given up active roles in clubs or spent less time outside home and work. Just under half had reduced physical activity — less sport, less exercise, less maintenance and repairs to house or car and less gardening. This last reduction in activity was considered very important, being often the first change to be mentioned; other members of the family were reported to have taken over, wives often cutting the grass and doing the digging; alternatively the problem had been solved by the purchase of a powered lawn-mower.

Very few, less than one in ten, had increased their social activities, although just under one quarter had increased their physical activity —

mostly walking and golf. This is one of the few indications that at
least a minority were following the more positive approach to
recovery which had been recommended. A few men who had
previously participated in more active sports such as tennis, skiing
and swimming and who gradually resumed their activities were, by
four years, back to their previous levels of activity, although sometimes
having abandoned competitive situations.

Some of those who had either reduced their activities or who had
never undertaken much leisure activity reported that they could do
little in the evening or weekends because they were exhausted after
a day's work. It is possible that the priority accorded to work means
that it is a fairly insensitive indicator of recovery and that reports of
successful outcome in terms of return to work may be obtained at the
expense of deterioration in other spheres of life.

Report on smoking habits showed considerable change from the
position at infarction. Most of this change appeared to have taken
place in the first twelve months after which the position had largely
stabilised. Only one man out of every eight was a non-smoker at
infarction but by twelve months the proportion of non-smokers had
increased to two out of every five and this remained the same at
four years (Table 13.10). Three out of every four men were in the two
heaviest smoking categories at infarction but only one in every four
at twelve months and this had declined slightly further to one in
every five at four years.

Changed expectations and roles within the family were reported
frequently, three out of every five men believing that they were now
treated in a different way by members of their family. Examples
included being expected to do less in the home, receiving more
consideration, not being pressed to undertake gardening or house
decoration and various responsibilities being taken over by other
members of the family. While these changes were designed by the
family members to be helpful, there was evidence that some of the
men considered that this role rearrangement had been carried to
excess since they felt capable of resuming many of their activities
and indeed these situations were a fairly common cause of family
conflict.

This contrasts with the work situation where a similar number,
two thirds, reported that rearrangements had been made for their
benefit but indicated that this help was appreciated. Sometimes this
had involved formal work rearrangement by the management or
informal reallocation by fellow employees. It was more often described

like this: 'If I need help with a heavy lift, I get it', 'the young lad
comes at once', or 'I get all the help I need.' Frequently the decision
to seek help was left to the man himself and appeared to be
fairly unobtrusive.

Such differences between reactions to adjustments at work and in
the home suggest that, in the structured work situation, ways had
been found, formal and informal, of negotiating change in a way which
avoided damaging the self-image of men who, as we have seen earlier,
were often very strongly oriented to instrumental roles. In contrast,
in families where, as we have already noted, both spouses often
appeared to lack ability in expressive roles, compensations less often
seemed to have emerged and there was evidence of failure to build
up a new self-image acceptable to both men and family members.

Men often appeared uncertain as to how the illness had affected
their families and although one in every three thought that the impact
had been very substantial, this would seem to underestimate the effect,
given the level of anxiety among wives at infarction and twelve months
later. It was, in fact, noticeable during the four year interviews with
the men that several wives appeared to be in poor health and there
were reports of others having been very ill at varying times; moreover
three wives themselves died in the interval between twelve months and
four years, all of coronary heart disease.

Attitudes

Although most men expressed complete satisfaction with their medical
care in both hospital and in the community, nearly one in every two
said that they felt they could have benefited from more advice on day-
to-day activities following discharge from hospital and indeed
throughout the months, and in some cases, years, that followed. Over
one third felt that they would have liked more opportunity to discuss
their illness and its implications with doctors and to learn more about
the condition. Sometimes this was to discuss points subsequently
raised by family, friends, workmates or the media (Table 13.11).

Such comments suggest that many 'flaws in the perception of
reality' may continue to exist because they are not seen as subjects
which may be appropriately raised with professionals. This is all the
more serious since there was still evidence of the existence of
considerable uncertainty and fear.

When men were asked if they felt that the illness was now quite
over, just under one third replied that they thought it was; an equal
number considered that it was not, while slightly over one third gave

variants indicating that the thought was always at the back of their minds.

Many people found it very difficult to decide if they had ever really got back to 'normal' and it seemed more meaningful to ask how long they felt it had taken to return to a reasonably stable way of living (Table 13.12). This was considered to have been achieved at four months after infarction by approximately one in every six, at nine months by over one third, at rather more than twelve months by one out of every five and at two years by one in every eight. The remainder, one in every six, felt that they had not achieved a state of stability at all.

No attempt was made to apply detailed attitude scales. Instead men were asked to comment both on how they now saw things in general and also what advice, based on their own experience, they would give to a friend who had just had an infarction. In reply two out of every three felt that they now looked at things differently, and half said that they considered all aspects of life more carefully. A smaller number were more specific, reporting that they were more concerned about their health; in particular these men tended to associate any symptom — any ache, pain or just a 'funny feeling' — with the heart or their illness, experiencing resultant anxiety or apprehension. Two out of every five felt deep concern about the way they were now limited, the things they could not do, and indeed would never do again. A sense of bereavement was manifest in allusions to many past activities — ranging from the ability to climb mountains and run for buses to matters of domestic and social routine.

The suddenness of onset appeared still to be of great significance to one out of every three. 'It couldn't have happened to me', 'I still don't really believe it', 'I had no warning.' In some cases, this suddenness of the original attack promoted a basis for continuing inactivity — 'It could happen again at any time.'

One of the areas where beliefs seemed to have changed is the association of factors with the onset of illness. Fewer people were sure that something in their way of life had been associated with the onset of the illness, although two out of every five still felt that the work situation had played some part. A few who indicated a specific factor, such as a source of stress in the family or work situation, felt reassured that this factor had now been removed or altered.

Overall, it was possible to detect three types of general response according to whether men expressed entirely positive attitudes, entirely negative attitudes, or a mixture. Typical of the first type of

response, expressed by approximately one quarter of the men, were
the following: 'Life is better', 'I am now happier', 'I am less easily
upset', 'I am more interested in life and other people', 'life is more
precious — it was a positive lesson for me', 'I knew I would be all
right from the beginning.'

A much larger group, rather more than half the total, expressed
only negative attitudes, of which the following were typical: 'I am
more easily upset', 'I worry more, I feel uncertain', 'I have lost
interest, life is worse', 'I worry about the future, it was a warning',
'I am much more concerned about my health', 'I have had my day, you
only get one chance, it could happen again', 'I feel I am not the man
I was.'

The first group appeared to have adopted from early days a
constructive, carefully planned approach to recovery, regarding the
illness as a learning experience and frequently commenting on the
improved quality of life. In contrast, the majority emphasised
negative aspects, deploring the ways in which their lives have become
limited and frequently expressed deep concern about the future.
Finally, there was another small group of approximately a quarter who
expressed a mixture of attitudes. Drawn from all these groups were
individuals, amounting to rather more than one quarter, who expressed
a real appreciation of being alive. They saw themselves as survivors;
the ones who were lucky, sometimes contrasting their good fortune
with someone whom they had known in hospital and who was now
dead.

Since such a large preponderance of negative attitudes persisted,
it is hardly surprising that few were able to suggest constructive 'recipes
for action' which they would recommend to a friend recovering from
a similar illness. The overriding consideration was generally to try to
provide reassurance, men sometimes indicating that this was because
of the fears and uncertainty which they had themselves experienced.
Half the men answered in terms of rather negative bromides such as
'don't worry', 'don't give in', 'forget about it', one third emphasised
the need to 'be careful', 'take it easy', another third (there was some
overlapping) echoed professional advice of a slightly more positive
character, mainly 'get back to normal'. Smaller numbers wanted to
give more specific positive advice such as 'get life organised', 'develop
new interests', 'take plenty of exercise', 'give up smoking' and 'don't
pay too much attention to doctors' instructions'.

Amongst the group who would prefer positive advice were those
who said they would point to their own experience — 'I have survived

and am making the most of life.' These appeared to be men of resource who would in fact have welcomed an opportunity to be involved in helping others, talking over their experiences with them and helping to overcome unnecessary fears and uncertainty in the early days of recovery. Apart from the positive stance of this minority (one in every four) most other advice appeared to be of the stereotyped kind which men had themselves received and which had proved of somewhat limited value to them.

14 STAGES AND UNDERLYING THEMES IN THE POST-INFARCTION CAREER

We have described in some detail several different aspects of the impact of myocardial infarction on a series of men and their wives. In this chapter we attempt to draw together the main themes which kept recurring in the definitions made both by men and by members of their families and social networks and, in particular, the key themes of fear and uncertainty which appeared to underly nearly all the most difficult contingencies encountered in recovery. In varying degrees these themes pervaded the various stages of the post-infarction career, making themselves manifest in changed self-images and roles, and all our evidence suggests that they present to professional services a challenge which has not yet been fully faced.

The application of the concept of 'career' to myocardial infarction patients proved to be particularly useful. This series of men could be seen starting on their post-infarction careers with the medical definition of having sustained a first infarction. For some there was a pre-infarction period of illness, in a few cases with recognised signs and symptoms of heart disease, but more frequently the symptoms were vague and ill-defined. For others the infarction was totally unexpected. After hospitalisation their experiences and time patterns varied widely, indicating the inadequacy of looking for any single point in time at which 'return to normality' can be expected.

Similarly, the concept 'definition of the situation' proved valuable in helping to understand the complexity of each patient's progress and changing attitudes over the months, and indeed years, following the attack. Emphasis on the patient as reacting, not just to the 'facts' of his illness, but to his perception of its implications, illuminated many of the misunderstandings which arose when his perception lacked congruence with definitions made by professionals or by 'significant others', especially wives.

The Post-Infarction Career

Although it is not possible to delineate a succession of clear-cut stages following one another at well defined intervals of time, never the less there appeared to be certain phases which were perceived by individuals as being of particular significance.

For most patients, the infarction itself is a *traumatic event* not easily forgotten by the man himself or by those with him when he often experienced severe pain, a sense of impending death and powerlessness to control events. There was for some a period ranging from several hours to several days of which they had little memory. Even at the beginning of the post-infarction career, many differences were apparent among those entering it; while some had previous experiences of other illnesses which had already modified their way of life, others had been suddenly transformed from a position of health and independence to one of totally unexpected life-threatening illness and total dependency on others. For most men the suddenness of the onset of the illness was of particular significance; they found it hard to believe that such a major discontinuity, with such profound implications, could have occurred in their lives. Most of them had known friends and relatives or had read about people who had experienced 'heart attacks' and many had some conception of what the illness meant in terms of severity, chance of dying and recovery. A few people, who experienced a gradual or mild onset and who carried on their regular activities for a few days, initially found it hard to accept that they were undergoing anything more than a trivial illness. For all of them infarction could hardly fail to be a landmark, if not a turning point in their health careers, their occupational careers and their family careers. Despite its great significance, this was, however, a very short stage and patients passed quickly into the second stage, taking the vivid memory of the traumatic event with them.

As we saw in Chapter 7, *the social space created by emergency hospitalisation* temporarily removes from patients the ability to make meaningful definitions of their individual situations and prospects; into this vacuum new and confusing definitions rush, initially the universally supported view that they are 'lucky to be alive' and that they must now 'obey doctors' orders'. In this new pattern of living the definitions made by family members and friends temporarily impinge less strongly than those made by staff and fellow patients.

As patients recover, they come to spend an increasing proportion of their time in observation of and interaction with the other patients. They soon discover which other patients are labelled as having the same illness — having perhaps even been admitted on the same day — and are able to compare treatment, progress, symptoms and dates of discharge. There were many indications in this series that contact with fellow patients at this period markedly affected the way in which some men come to see their own illness, sometimes contributing to

considerable changes of mood. Although slightly longer than the
previous stage, this also is now a short period of time (although,
quite recently, when total inactivity and prolonged bed rest were part
of the routine treatment this must have been a much longer period of
great uncertainty). With rapid mobilisation and emphasis on active
approach to recovery, most patients, apart from those with a very
severe infarction, or with a complication, move quickly into the next
stage leaving behind these marked fluctuations in mood.

Towards the end of their stay in hospital there comes a *time of
optimism* for most patients. Having emerged from a dreadful
experience, men in this series began to feel 'more like themselves';
pain had gone, appetite was restored, encouraging comments about
their progress and appearance were made by staff and visitors, they
were able to move around the ward, often noting that other patients
appeared in worse condition than themselves, and they were preparing
either to go straight home or to spend a short time in a convalescent
hospital. Many were making hopeful and confident definitions of the
future (anticipating fewer problems than their wives admitted to in
separate interviews); indeed half the men were quite emphatic that
there would be no problems and fewer than one in ten expressed
serious worries. Visits from colleagues or employers confirming that
their job was waiting for them and that they need have no worries
on that score were very reassuring in instances where there had
initially been uncertainty about the security of employment.

Although for some, this mood of optimism and confidence
continues, leading smoothly towards recovery, *the immediate post-
hospital phase opens up considerable differences between patients
and brings to many a pronounced sense of depression, anxiety or
frustration*, previous fears and uncertainties being reactivated and new
ones arising. Many men reported that they had not realised how weak
they were at the time of discharge nor how easily tired they would be.
They found that they could be readily defeated when attempting
tasks demanding relatively little mental or physical activity. There
were complaints about lack of information on what they could and
could not do and as to when they could resume activities such as
sexual intercourse and car driving. They found difficulty in
communicating with doctors, especially over matters which they
regarded as important but which many felt were considered to be
trivial or irrelevant by the doctor. Without adequate support and
advice there is a danger that symptoms, which for many are a normal
part of early recovery, persist much longer and interfere with the later

stages of recovery.

The period which follows is generally one of *assessment and adjustment*. This is a time when the numerous factors which may effect outcome come under consideration. Some of these factors may well have been operative long before the infarction. Many men spoke of looking back and trying to find a cause for the illness or at least something which may have contributed towards it. Their beliefs about causation often reflected common lay conceptions, particularly the idea of excessive work as being a strain or social life being too stressful.

Six months after the illness there was still considerable evidence of disturbance to the quality of life in all spheres. Many patients spoke of continued uncertainty as to what they were able to do. Many also were emphatic that there were continuing social, personal and occupational problems and that they did not see the illness as over. Fears were often expressed, usually of recurrence of a heart attack or about their ability to cope in the future and complaints about difficulties in adaptation were frequent.

This period of transition leads on to a *gradual normalisation process* which may last several years. Changes seen were sometimes incremental in character, involving, for instance, deliberately and consistently taking more exercise or planning more positively for leisure time; sometimes, there was a process of substitution, for instance, a change in diet, different work or a switch from team sports to non-competitive or individual types of physical recreation; most frequently, however, changes involved decrease — cutting down of social and physical activities, reduction in hours of work or in responsibilities and attempts to reduce weight or smoking.

Role Loss, Identity Crisis, Fear and Uncertainty

Elements of role loss or role diminution appear to be reflected in a crisis of identity which occurs for many patients at varying times in the post-infarction career, when they feel that they are no longer the person whom they have been. The illness seemed to raise for many men in this series fundamental questions about the nature of their being, their abilities and their future. In particular the male role as a strong, independent, virile husband and father, responsible as chief breadwinner in the family and capable of solving his own problems, appeared to be called into question to a greater extent than is the case in most other illnesses. This identity crisis has to be resolved by a process in which a new self-image is gradually built up in interaction

with significant others. For some men in this series the process was
a painful and negative one, leaving a lasting feeling of 'no longer being
the man I was' or of 'being thrown on the scrap-heap'.

Underlying this identity crisis and loss of role can be seen interlocked
elements of fear and uncertainty. Although the intensity diminishes
throughout the recovery period, never the less, even four years after
the infarction, and even in men who have had no further episodes of
illness and who appear to have made a very satisfactory recovery, there
was at least the hint of fear of a further attack. Virtually all patients
knew someone who had a recurrence and someone who had died
after a further attack. Sometimes the fear was predominantly of
recurrence, often being related back to the frightening nature of the
attack which they had experienced: 'I couldn't go through that
again.' Sometimes fear was mainly of pain or of being unable to
function normally in a work or social situation. Many of these fears
tended to persist. As one man put it — 'the thought is always with
you. I don't tell anybody. I don't want to think about it.'

The existence of such fears, especially where they were not
acknowledged, inevitably contributed to uncertainty about what
should and what should not be done. This was compounded where
medical advice was seen to be vague or conflicting. Comments like
'don't get too tired', 'take it easy', 'learn your limitations', 'take more
exercise', 'don't worry', 'be careful', can only produce uncertainty,
confusion and conflict. They can be interpreted differently by patient
and family and may appear quite unrelated to individual situations as
defined by patients and their families. There was evidence of
considerable discontinuity between the avowed professional aim of
'return to normality by three or six months', and the actual practical
advice given to the patient. This is the more confusing if there have also
been questions or comments which imply that some aspect of his
normal way of life — work, leisure, smoking or eating habits — may
have been in some way associated with the onset of illness.

Contrasting Careers: 'Room to Manoeuvre'

Lack of sustained professional help geared to their individual needs
on such key issues can leave patients in a state of dissonance which,
as Festinger[1] has shown, is psychologically uncomfortable. In
attempting to reduce this dissonance their own social and psychological
resources and those of their network members become correspondingly
important.

In this respect the contrasting careers and outcomes seen in this series point to the importance of 'room to manoeuvre' both in economic and emotional terms. Men in certain non-manual occupations (such as the professions, self-employment of a prosperous nature or work for a firm that was strongly oriented to welfare provision) had advantages in being able to see role change at work in more positive terms, e.g. finding satisfaction in giving responsibility and scope to juniors; such men often had access to compensatory roles in family and community, enabling them to build up different, but enhanced, self-images. They also tended to have been, already before infarction, more active, both mentally and physically, than most. A few other men, utilising the occasion to reassess their way of life, found something unsatisfactory in one or more roles and made carefully planned changes. As noted in Chapter 8, one such was the salesman whose wife felt that he would never have had the confidence to change to training for clerical work if he had not been forced into recognising that he must abandon his stressful occupation. Men who made such changes were particularly prone to comment on their greater appreciation of life and its improved quality.

They were, however, very much in the minority. More often, men seemed to feel constrained either by economic circumstances or by their own health or personality or a combination of these: changes in roles were in a negative direction and no compensatory gains appeared feasible. This applied particularly among manual workers as well as among non-manual men who were either in self-employment of a financially insecure type or in highly competitive commercial or industrial employment.

As we saw in Chapter 9, many such men appeared to find the 'burden of explanation' weighing heavily on them and this could deter them from embarking on new activities and exploring new roles. Furthermore, they appeared to have previously been intensively committed to instrumental roles and lacking ability in expressive ones.

It was often the wives of just these men who appeared particularly at a loss as to how to help their husbands; the resignation with which many anticipated their husband's inability to adapt seemed to be an indication of some degree of atrophy in emotional relations in the family, pointing to the need for skilled help to be offered to wives as well as husbands. Moreover it was also often such women, who, as we saw in Chapter 12, seemed isolated or restricted in the sources of informal emotional support available to them.

For these reasons we think that the widely different types of outcome experienced by men in this series have implications for other patients — both men and women — and for their families as well as for those planning and operating rehabilitation services. Increased awareness of the range of difficulties likely to arise in recovery and the possibility of identifying many of these at an early stage should enable professionals to adapt advice and services more closely to individual needs.

Notes

1. Festinger, L. (1962). *A Theory of Cognitive Dissonance*, London, Tavistock.

15 IMPLICATIONS FOR POLICY : CRISIS EQUALS 'DANGER' PLUS 'OPPORTUNITY'

As has been found in other studies, noted in earlier chapters, severity of infarction did not appear to be a sufficient determinant of outcome of this series. Nor, since services after leaving hospital were so little used, can differential utilisation of formal rehabilitation facilities be considered of main significance. Instead, we found differences in outcome more often to be associated with the nature and extent of concurrent physical, social and psychological problems facing men and their families and the resources which were available within themselves and in their informal social networks to help them cope.

We think that the contrasting experiences which they encountered have implications for policy and planning in health, social and educational services. There appears to be an assumption in the medical profession that the majority of men are little affected by a first myocardial infarction and consequently that rehabilitation services are not particularly appropriate or important after this illness. It may be, however, that the experience of those who *are* little affected has been too easily accepted as standard, perhaps partly because such men are often in non-manual occupations and thus more 'visible,' frequently being known socially to members of the medical profession. This encourages medical advice to remain geared to the needs of the executive stereotype — cutting down on committees, keeping up of golf — so that the different social and psychological problems increasingly besetting younger men, manual workers and those with other intercurrent illnesses or difficulties are insufficiently recognised.

There are also official and professional pressures towards playing down ill effects less employees should be discouraged and lest patients become cardiac neurotics'. While recognising that these can be dangers, we think that current emphasis on the concept of 'return to normality' may well serve to conceal the very real problems encountered by many men and their families particularly because it seems to belittle the degree of adaptation which may be required. It also assumes that the 'normality' existing before the illness represents a satisfactory situation to which to return.

Failure by professional services to recognise the full implications of rehabilitation needs after myocardial infarction and to think through the range of contingencies confronting individual patients in widely differing social settings may leave patients and families in a stage of chronic role conflict. The post-infarction career becomes all too easily a series of 'double bind' situations in which, on the one hand, patients are expected to 'get back to normal' and, on the other, to accept that one or more features of their normal way of life (for instance, smoking, obesity, overwork, worrying) is harmful.

In particular, we found evidence of failure in communication between patients and general practitioners. A few doctors were felt to be like 'friends of the family' but many were seen as lacking insight into problems particularly those relating to patients' personalities, family relationships and work. It may be that many doctors, consciously or unconsciously, are at a loss because medical education in the past has not equipped them to understand the life-styles of many patients, particularly when these are younger men or when they belong to lower social classes. Some of these deficiencies may be expected to be remedied in the future as a result of the introduction of behavioural sciences into the undergraduate curriculum of most medical schools, provided that, as we have argued elsewhere,[1] these subjects are made clearly relevant to concurrent experience with patients in diverse family and community settings and that opportunities are also provided for students to learn from the different perspectives of professionals and lay workers in para-medical and non-medical services. In the meantime there is considerable need for the expansion of post-graduate courses in these subjects.

It may also be that many doctors expect — as did many wives — that 'nothing can be done' and that most post-infarction patients cannot or will not change their life-styles. They overlook the evidence that such pessimistic interpretations are not accepted so readily in some other situations where psychiatric, educational or guidance counselling, sustained if necessary over time, has been found to help individuals and their families towards a clearer awareness of their needs and gradual working through of modifications of attitudes and behaviour.

For reasons such as these many doctors, while accepting the new and more positive approach in physical rehabilitation, tend to limit themselves to the medical model, shying away from psycho-social approaches as outside their province. We think that a more appropriate model would be to see the post-infarction career as a psycho-social transition, parallel to that following many other illnesses, in which patients and families could be helped towards acknowledging the need

to adapt and using the opportunity to move towards greater maturity.
Parkes[2] described as a common problem in such transitions 'the
tendency to maintain the *status quo* at all costs and to avoid learning
the tasks appropriate to a new, unwanted world'.

As an illustration relating to another type of handicap, Parkes
quotes the contention of Fitzgerald[3] that partial blindness may be
more of a disability than complete blindness because it encourages
the blind person to continue to function as if he could see instead of
learning the skills appropriate to blindness. Parkes adds that:

> those who are in a position to give support and guidance at such
> times must be prepared to assist the other person to examine his
> assumptions, to clarify the model of the world which predated the
> transition and the situation which now obtains in order to discover
> what aspects of it must change and which aspects can be retained.
> Although this is a painful and time-consuming business and requires
> of the helper patience, tact and understanding, it is also extremely
> rewarding work, leading, as it usually does, to very obvious
> improvement in the competence and morale of the person who is
> changing.

Without pushing the parallel too far, this type of approach seems
to have implications for myocardial infarction in that, during the
post-infarction career, individuals may look unchanged and function
normally within limits but may maintain assumptions inappropriate
to these limitations.

Similarly, approaches to psycho-social change which have been
evolved in therapeutic communities for the rehabilitation of addicts
and in organisations like Alcoholics Anonymous and Gamblers
Anonymous may also have implications in the combination of self-help
and sustained support which they offer. It may be argued against this
that such social crutches are needed only by those perceived to be
the 'weaker' members of the community — those who succumb to
afflictions like mental illness or addictions which still often carry
stigma. In contrast to such conditions, coronary heart disease carries
stigma only occasionally (when it can be ascribed to a reprehensible
personality trait, as when a woman in this series blamed it on her
husband's ill-temper with their son). Usually, coronary patients are
seen as respectable, strong, capable persons; where failings are
detected they are often seen as virtues carried to excess — overwork,
perfectionism. The price of being respected rather than stigmatised

may be not to be offered the social crutches which have helped others recovering from less 'respectable' afflictions. At the same time patients may be expected to have sufficient 'will-power' to withdraw without support from long-term dependence on personal crutches such as smoking or overeating.

Mechanic[4] has suggested that patients recovering from mental illness sometimes need to learn the coping skills required in interpersonal negotiation as part of the process of substituting an educational model for the medical model in rehabilitation. Many of his suggestions appear applicable to the post-infarction career, especially since he draws particular attention to the needs of patients from impoverished social environments. Although only a minority of men in this series were impoverished in material terms at the time of the study, there were indications, discussed in earlier chapters, that many more had endured considerable early deprivation in their families of origin and we have suggested that this may have failed to prepare them for the type of life-style and the stage in the family life cycle which they had reached at the time of infarction.

Among the skills advocated by Mechanic the following seem particularly apposite : initiating new relationships; developing alternative social relationships; distributing interpersonal investments against the threat of loss; handling hostility and aggression through humour; techniques of interpersonal trading and compromise; learning to keep interpersonal channels open and yet protect oneself simultaneously. As Mechanic points out, professional workers themselves are not yet used to thinking about behaviour in this way and a good deal more work is required to describe more adequately these subtle but important interpersonal skills and to try putting this educational model into practice.

A few experiments in the use of group therapy after myocardial infarction are currently being tried in a number of countries and we think that they could be extended. Such settings can provide opportunities for practice in the development of the interpersonal skills advocated by Mechanic. By introducing new 'significant others' to patients they could also be seen as an effective way of strengthening social networks where these are identified as being deficient in constructive support. Family members and friends could also be involved, sometimes in joint sessions and other times separately.

Objection is sometimes made to the possible use of group therapy on the grounds that if a patient were to die while the group was still in being this might have a disturbing effect on the remaining members. It may be, however, that this experience could be more constructively accepted if discussed within a therapeutic community of fellow sufferers rather than when learned from a newspaper at home. Several wives reported husbands being upset by receiving news of the death of a former fellow patient and it seemed likely that others had similarly heard such news without having felt able to talk through the emotions aroused.

We think it important that participation should not be limited to patients whose illnesses begin concurrently but should be extended to draw on the resources of former patients who have made favourable adjustments, as well as some of their relatives and friends. The co-operation of knowledgeable volunteers has been drawn on for many years in some specialised rehabilitation services, two outstanding examples involving patients who have undergone colostomy and amputations. We suggest that such schemes could usefully be extended to other rehabilitation services including recovery from myocardial infarction. Several patients when seen at four years expressed a wish to participate in this way. Such schemes might most easily be organised within a general practice setting but might also in some circumstances be based on the larger hospital practices. The emphasis which we have placed here on the use of psycho-therapy and socio-therapy should not be taken to entail neglect of physical factors in rehabilitation. Goal-setting techniques, similar to those advocated for other disabilities by Kushlick and his colleagues,[5] would seem to be particularly applicable to modification of exercise, diet and smoking habits and could fit well with the approach which we suggest.

Although we have emphasised how little use was made of professional services other than the hospital and the general practitioner and have pointed to deficiences in the quality of communication with the latter, we are not suggesting that there should be a further proliferation of professionals but rather that more effective use should be made of existing services and that they should be integrated with the resources and goodwill that exist among lay members of the community.

This would involve a new approach to team care in the community and we suggest that there is room for experiment in different ways of organising this, all aiming at encouraging professionals from different specialisms to bring together their skills and learn from each other in an interdisciplinary setting. Action research projects, carefully evaluated, should seek early identification of patients most likely to be at risk, in terms of their total social situation as well as their physical and psychiatric status. Social workers and health visitors, both in hospital and general practice settings, could receive more encouragement to participate in such action research. Various ways of assessing outcome could be tried, using, as we have attempted, subjective as well as objective criteria.

A constructive example of the interdisciplinary approach is to be seen in work undertaken in Edinburgh on a larger series than ours by Cay and her colleagues.[6,7] Cay's perspective, as a psychiatrist, leads her to conclusions which fit well with those induced by our perspective from medical sociology. Her most recent study[8] shows the possibilities of combining social work intervention with ready access to psychiatric support when this is required.

Our own experience in the fields of community and occupational medicine has led us to make a plea for recognition of the important part that nurses can play in the team outside the hospital. One such role is in the community in the early stages of recovery working with patient and family, helping to mediate the transition from hospital to general practitioner. Anther role is in the work situation, where a nurse trained in occupational health can provide support carefully adapted to individual needs, often being in a better position to establish day-to-day relationships with fellow-employees and sometimes more alert to likely problems in the specific work situation than a doctor even if the latter is also trained in occupational health.

In addition to more positive action by employment services and employers, there is a need for increased provision of sheltered workshops as well as opportunities for home occupational therapy and voluntary community service for men who cannot return to work, who might regain some sense of role if they could participate in an organisation which made demands on their former skills or encouraged the development of new interests. This requires imaginative and flexible types of co-operation between statutory services, voluntary organisations and community enterprises. There are signs that workers in community education may in future be able to contribute a more flexible approach where older services may have become unduly compartmentalised and restricted.

Such new approaches to team care and self-care within the community imply the need for the acceptance of a 'learning model' as being appropriate to the recovery process. Some degree of uncertainty and limitation must remain after even the most seemingly successful short-term recovery. The experiences of this series of men suggest that acceptance of such uncertainty and limitation can best be met by facing the need for building new self-images and new assumptive worlds.

The word 'crisis' is formed in Chinese of two ideograms, the first meaning 'danger,' the second 'opportunity.' Perhaps Western medicine concentrates services unduly on the first part and neglects the second. In this series those men who were able to see the crisis as an opportunity needed little professional support because they already had sufficient potential resources in themselves and in their social networks. Where, however, such resources were lacking, professional services also appeared to be deficient.

The principles of modern rehabilitation require a progressive handing back of responsibility for self-care to the patient. In practice, it is not sufficiently often realised that two corollaries are entailed: understanding by professionals of the total social situation of individual patients and readiness on the part of doctors themselves to learn new roles so that they come to be seen as 'learning resources' rather than as authoritarian figures whose edicts may be forgotten or circumvented but never questioned nor discussed. If, in the event, doctors are not willing to enlarge their roles in this way, they may prefer to share the 'learning resources' role with other agencies in the community. Appositely, there would appear to be scope in the expanding field of adult education, where emphasis is turning towards community participation in educational programmes, and also in new developments within the health education component of the reorganised health service.

Changes in the direction which we have suggested would amount to an admission by health and social services that mere survival is not enough and that more positive intervention is needed to help many survivors and their families work towards a more satisfactory quality of life. This would present services with an immense challenge, given the increasing incidence of coronary heart disease and its advance into younger age groups and all social classes. The quality of care at the emergency created by myocardial infarction is already recognised as important, although expensive in the services required; one could argue that it is, at the very least, wasteful not to look ahead to developing more effective and more sustained services for survivors, which might also minimise readmissions. Overall costs should not thereby be increased, especially if, as we have argued, use were to be made of volunteer help emerging from among former patients and their families.

There may be more general implications. We have suggested that parallels exist between the needs of post-infarction patients and those recovering from mental illness and various forms of addiction. If the rehabilitation services which are required after such different types of crisis are seen to involve similar processes — in particular, the learning of new roles and the practice of interpersonal skills within a better informed community of present and past fellow patients, drawing on but not over-dependent on professional help — does not this point also to the need for a similar interdisciplinary approach to the prevention of this and other diseases with a stress component? If the different professionals set themselves systematically to learn from their patients' experiences, to pool the insights thus gained and then to feed them back into the community through educational channels, as well as through medical and social services, might this not reduce vulnerability to some other kinds of illness as well as coronary heart disease?

Notes

1. McEwen, J. and Finlayson, A. (1975). A Medical Sociology Course in a Revised Curriculum. *British Journal of Medical Education* 9, 236-43.
2. Parkes, C.M. (1972). What Becomes of Redundant World Models? A Contribution to the Study of Adaptation to Change. Paper presented at Third International Conference on Social Science and Medicine, Elsinore. Mimeographed.
3. Fitzgerald, R. (1970). Reactions to Blindness. An Exploratory Study of Adults with Recent Loss of Sight. *Archives of General Psychiatry* 22, 370-9.
4. Mechanic, D. (1968) *Medical Sociology*, New York, Free Press.
5. Kushlick, A., Blunden, R., Horner, D., Smith, J. Goal-setting. (1975). In: *The Handicapped Person in the Community* (Unit 9), Milton Keynes, Open University Press.
6. Cay, E.L., Vetter, N., Philips, A.E., Dugard, P. (1972). Psychological Status during Recovery from an Acute Heart Attack. *Journal of Psychosomatic Research* 16, 425-35.
7. Cay, E.L., Vetter, N. Philips, A.E. (1973). Practical Aspects of Cardiac Rehabilitation: Psycho-social factors. *Giornale Italiano di Cardiologia*, 3 646-55.
8. Cay, E.L. (1975). Rehabilitation after a Heart Attack. The Team Approach. *Proceedings of the Third International College of Psychosomatic Medicine*, Rome.

APPENDIX

Table 1: Men who died before twelve months: Age by social class

Age	Non-manual	Manual
-39	1	0
40-44	1	2
45-49	1	0
50-54	0	2
55-59	0	5
	3	9

Table 2: Men who died before twelve months: 'Areas of potential stress' assessed

Number of areas assessed as of potential stress	Number of families
0-2 areas	2
3-5 areas	10

Individual areas of potential stress	Non-manual	Manual	All
Man's pre-infarction health	2	6	8
Man's work	0	4	4
Man's personality	3	6	9
Nuclear family	2	9	11
Network	1	7	8

Table 3: Men who died before twelve months: Smoking habits

MRC Smoking Category	Husband	Wife
1) Non smoker	3	7
2) Moderate	1	0
3)	2	4
4) Heavy	5	1
5)	1	0

Table 4.1: Health before infarction (100% = 78)

(a)   17% had symptoms which had been recognised as evidence of heart disease.

of these { 10% knew they had angina
{ 7% had other symptoms most often related to hypertension

of these { 9% had experienced symptoms for more than 1 year
{ 3% had experienced symptoms for more than 1 month but less than 1 year
{ 5% had experienced symptoms for more than 1 day but less than 1 month

(b)   53% claimed that they had generally been feeling unwell.

of these { 13% had experienced symptoms for more than 1 year
{ 19% had experienced symptoms for more than 1 month but less than 1 year
{ 21% had experienced symptoms for more than 1 day but less than 1 month

(c)   31% had been attending their general practitioners the few weeks prior to infarction.

(d)   23% described themselves as currently ill.

(e)   8% claimed to have a history of frequent and/or severe illness in the past.

Notes: (i) First Interviews: 78 men were seen but only 76 wives. This accounts for different totals in tables.
(ii) DK = Do not know
NA = Not applicable or Not asked

Table 4.2: Onset of illness (100% = 78)

(a) Place Where Onset Occurred

Home	58%
Work	15%
Elsewhere	27%
	(100%)

(b) Activity When Onset Occurred

Resting (Sitting or Sleeping)	44%
Active	50%
Very Active	6%
	(100%)

(c) Circumstances When Onset Occurred

With Family	71%
With Friends (including Workmates)	9%
With Strangers	1%
Alone	19%
	(100%)

(d) Medical Advice at Time of Onset (before admission to Hospital)

Seen by Own General Practitioner	67%
Seen by Other Doctor	6%
Not Seen by Doctor	27%
	(100%)

Table 4.3: Time interval between onset of symptoms and admission to hospital (100% = 78)[*]

$<$1 hour	30%
1-2 hours	19%
2-3 hours	8%
3-5 hours	17%
5-10 hours	6%
10-24 hours	6%
$>$ 24 hours	13%
	(99%)

---

[*]approximate time intervals were used as few patients or their wives remembered exact times.

Table 5.1: Occupational Background (100% = 78)

(a)   Employment

Working Prior to infarction	94%
Unemployed	5%
Currently Off Sick	1%
	(100%)

(b)   Occupational Changes During Preceding 5 years (more than one change is possible)

54% had experienced no major changes in occupation.

While:—

31% had changed employer

22% had changed status in their employment

9% had changed nature of their work

8% had frequent changes

(c)   Attitudes to Work

14% felt that they were not physically fit enough to do their work properly.

14% felt that they had some difficulties with their work.

17% were not completely happy with their work.

6% stated that they were unhappy or had difficulties with their fellow workers.

Table 5.2: Main Study Population: Age and Social Class Distribution (100% = 76)

Age		All	Non-manual	Manual
	-39	5 (7%)	2 (7%)	3 (6%)
	40-44	8 (11%)	1 (4%)	7 (15%)
	45-49	21 (28%)	8 (29%)	13 (27%)
	50-54	21 (28%)	8 (29%)	13 (27%)
	55-59	21 (28%)	9 (32%)	12 (25%)
	Total	76 (100%)	28 (100%)	48 (100%)

Note: Tables 5.6, 5.10 and 5.11
   * based on husband's occupation

Table 5.3: Housing

House:	Non-manual %	Manual %	All %	
Owner Occupied	40	8	20	
Privately Rented	7	15	12	
Council	53	77	68	(n=76)

Table 5.4: Transport

Car/Motorcycle:	Non-manual %	Manual %	All %	
Owned	86	67	74	
Not Owned	14	33	26	(n=76)

Table 5.5: Telephone

Telephone:	Non-manual %	Manual %	All %	
Installed	71	32	46	
Not Installed	29	68	54	(n=76)

Table 5.6: Geographical Origin

	Men			Women *		
	Non-manual	Manual	All	Non-Manual	Manual	All
	%	%	%	%	%	%
Incomers						
Long Distance						
(from outside Scotland)	10	3	5	14	4	8
Medium Distance						
(Scotland, Not Near)	7	8	8	11	17	14
Short Distance						
(Neighbouring County)	25	12	17	29	12	18
Sedentes						
Born Dundee City	50	66	61	43	58	53
Born Neighbouring						
Small Town/Village	7	10	9	3	8	7
						(n=76)

Table 5.7: Denomination of Origin

	Husband		Wife	
	Remaining	Changed	Remaining	Changed
	%	%	%	%
Church of Scotland	59	7	62	5
Roman Catholic	18	0	18	5
Church of England/Other	12	4	7	3
	89	11	87	13
				(n=76)

Table 5.8: Father's Occupation (Registrar General's Classification)

	Husband	Wife	
	%	%	
I and II	22	14	
IIIa	1	8	
III	26	29	
IV and V	50	46	
DK/NA	0	3	(n=76)

Table 5.9: Parents Available

	Husband		Wife	
	Father	Mother	Father	Mother
	%	%	%	%
Alive, locally available	14	22	17	36
Alive, not locally available	3	9	12	13
Died when subject under 15	17	13	16	11
Died in last 2 years	7	3	1	5
Died, other	59	53	54	36
				(n=76)

Table 5.10: Size of Family of Origin

	Husband			Wife*		
	Non-manual	Manual	All	Non-manual	Manual	All
	%	%	%	%	%	%
Size one	3	4	7	4	4	8
Size two	3	4	7	9	8	17
Size three	13	14	28	5	8	13
Size four	4	11	14	7	21	28
Size five to seven	9	21	30	3	17	20
Size eight plus	5	9	14	9	5	14
	37	63	100	37	63	100
						(n=76)

Table 5.11: Members of Family of Origin Still Available Locally

	Husband			Wife*		
	Non-manual	Manual	All	Non-manual	Manual	All
	%	%	%	%	%	%
At least one	50	75	66	54	77	62
None	50	25	33	46	23	32
						(n=76)

Table 5.12: Adult Children in Family

	Non-manual	Manual	All
	%	%	%
None over 16	12	12	24
At least one over 16	25	51	76
	37	63	100
			(n=76)

Table 5.13: Wives' Paid Employment

	Husband		
	Non-manual	Manual	All
	%	%	%
None	50	24	33
Normally full-time	25	40	34
Normally part-time	25	35	33
			(n=76)

Table 5.14: Wives' Health

	Husband		
	Non-manual	Manual	All
	%	%	%
Consulted GP	50	72	64
Ill, no consultation	10	8	9
No illness	39	18	26
			(n=76)

Table 5.15: Number of Areas of Potential Stress

	Husband		
	Non-manual	Manual	All
	%	%	%
0 - 2	50	29	37
3 - 5	50	71	63
			(n=76)

Table 6.1: Relationship between wife's expectations and husbands' occupation

Wife's expectations favourable about:—	Husbands' Occupation			
	I,II,IIIa %	III %	IV,V %	All %
Work	55	51	18	44
Exercise	71	69	68	69
Smoking (will stop)	(32)	(26)	(14)	(25)
Smoking (non-smoker)	(23)	(6)	(14)	(14)
Smoking combined	55	31	28	39
Consulting Doctor	87	46	55	63
Money	77	57	23	57
Difficulties (husband)	57	34	18	36
Difficulties (self)	29	20	18	23
(n =	31	35	22	88)

Table 6.2: Relationship between wife's expectation and husbands' age.

Wife's expectations favourable about:—	Husbands' Age				
	-44 %	45-49 %	50-54 %	55-59 %	All %
Work	29	50	52	42	44
Exercise	53	68	74	77	69
Smoking (will stop)					(25)
Smoking (non-smoker)					(14)
Smoking combined	12	32	61	42	39
Consulting Doctor	65	59	61	65	63
Money	59	77	48	42	57
Difficulties (husband)	24	36	43	38	36
Difficulties (self)	18	32	22	19	23
(n =	17	22	23	26	88)

Table 7.1: Men's beliefs as to factors associated with onset of illness
(100% = 78)

Factors related to their Work	40%
Factors related to their Leisure Activities	12%
Factors related to their Smoking	8%
Factors related to their Other Activities	24%

41% had no beliefs as to associated factors.

Table 7.2 Treatment following discharge from hospital

(a)   Drug Treatment (not including Anticoagulants)   (100%=78)

	At Discharge	Three Months	Six Months
YES	79%	78%	65%
NO	21%	22%	35%
	(100%)	(100%)	(100%)

(b)   Number of Drugs taken by those on Treatment at Discharge (100%=62)

1 drug	34%
2 drugs	22%
3 drugs	25%
4 drugs	17%
5 drugs	2%
	(100%)

Table 7.3: Contact with medical services (100%=78)

(a)   Attendance at Hospital Outpatient Clinics (excluding Anticoagulant Clinic)

Number of visits during six months following discharge.

NONE	23%
1	29%
2	19%
3	13%
4	5%
5	3%
6	8%
	(100%)

(b)   Contact with general practitioner

Number of visits during six months following discharge (excluding collection of repeat prescriptions when no contact with Doctor)

	At Home	At Surgery
None	52%	4%
1	16%	4%
2	8%	9%
3	6%	11%
4	5%	27%
5	4%	10%
6	5%	15%
7		5%
8	3%	4%
9		1%
10 or more	1%	10%
	(100%)	(100%)

Table 7.4: Summary of subject areas on which patients remembered receiving information and/or advice (100%=78)

	In Hospital	From GP	Both	Neither	Not Applicable
Smoking	25%	3%	50%	8%	14%
Diet	22%	13%	25%	40%	—
Exercise	22%	13%	45%	20%	—
Time of Return to Work	20%	22%	36%	22%	—
Social Activities	28%	8%	4%	60%	—
Personal Activities	17%	3%	3%	77%	—
Car Driving	35%	9%	9%	27%	20%

Table 8.1: Return to Work — Anticipation of difficulties while in hospital (100%=78)

No worries about return to work	50%
Specific difficulties anticipated	35%
General anxiety about return to work	15%
	(100%)
Threatened with redundancy	21%

Table 8.2: Return to work — Summary of position at six months

| | Outcome Successful | | | Outcome Not Successful | |
	Returned to Former Employment	Working in Different Employment	Retraining	Retired	Not Working
Overall	72%	5%	1%	3%	19%
Severity					
Mild	76%	6%	—	—	18%
Moderate	76%	5%	3%	3%	13%
Severe	61%	4%	—	4%	30%
Social Class					
I and II	83%	—	—	4%	13%
III(a)	71%	—	14%	—	14%
III(b)	77%	10%	—	3%	10%
IV and V	47%	6%	—	—	47%
Age					
-39	60%	—	20%	—	20%
40-44	44%	11%	—	—	44%
45-49	82%	9%	—	—	9%
50-54	81%	5%	—	—	14%
55-59	67%	—	—	10%	24%

Table 8.3: Return to work — advice received (100% = 78)

	In Hospital	From General Practitioner
Specific	19%	23%
General	32%	53%
None	47%	13%
Not Applicable (not yet fit for work)	2%	11%
	(100%)	(100%)

16% were advised a permanent change of occupation.

28% were advised a temporary change at time of return to work.

9% were advised to have a trial at former employment.

Table 8.4: Modification of work following infarction — position at six months (100% = 60)

(a) OVERALL — Hours of work

Reduced hours of work	45%
Same hours of work	48%
Increased hours of work	7%
	(100%)

(b) Hours of work — related to nature of previous employment

Light work	24% had decreased hours of work
Moderate work	52% had decreased hours of work
Heavy work	63% had decreased hours of work

(c) Overall modification of work related to severity of infarction

	Work Modified	
SEVERITY	NO	YES
Mild	8%	15%
Moderate	17%	35%
Severe	8%	17%
	(100%)	

Table 8.5: Difficulties following return to work — position at six months (100% = 60)

No difficulties at all	28%
Difficulties initially not serious	33%
Difficulties initially only but serious	8%
Continuing intermittent difficulties	13%
Serious continuing difficulties	12%
Difficulties resulting in giving up employment	5%
	(99%)

Table 9.1: Presence of symptoms after infarction (100% = 78)

	3 months	6 months
Angina	51%	51%
Other (related to heart)	39%	38%
No symptoms	24%	25%

Note: Some patients experienced angina and other symptoms.

Table 9.2: Participation in activities after infarction — position at six months (100% = 78)

	Physical Activities	Social Activities
Less	41%	37%
Same (reasonably active)	16%	29%
Same (never did much)	28%	31%
More	15%	3%
	(100%)	(100%)

Table 9.3: Smoking Patterns (100% = 78)

(a)   Before Infarction (Pipe and Cigars converted to cigarette equivalents 9% of total)

Non-smoker	Ex-smoker	10-14/day	15-24/day	25-49/day	50 or more/day
5%	11%	17%	29%	33%	5%

(b)   After Infarction

Percentage of smokers who succeeded in stopping smoking

At discharge	63%
At 3 months	38%
At 6 months	34%

Percentage stopped smoking by age

− 44 years	8%
45-54 years	46%
55-59 years	30%

Percentage stopped smoking by social class

I, II, III	40%
IV, V	17%

Smoking habits at 6 months compared with before illness

Stopped	34%
Decreased	46%
Same	14%
Increased	6%
	(100%)

Table 9.4 Men: Pre-infarction Smoking Patterns

MRC Categories*		All	Occupational Non-manual	Manual	Age —44	45-54	55+
			%	%	%	%	%
Category 1	non-smoker	12	18	8	0	12	19
Category 2	moderate	4	11	0	8	0	10
Category 3		11	14	8	0	12	14
Category 4	heavy	39	36	42	38	48	22
Category 5		34	21	42	54	29	33
(n =		76	28	48	13	42	21)

*Wives' definitions used.

Table 9.5 Women: Smoking Patterns Before and After Husbands' Infarction

MRC Categories*		BEFORE All	Occupation Non-manual	Manual	AFTER All	Occupation Non-manual	Manual
		%	%	%	%	%	%
Category 1	non-smoker	46	61	38	51	61	46
Category 2	moderate	12	11	13	7	11	4
Category 3		16	11	19	16	7	21
Category 4	heavy	20	11	25	20	14	23
Category 5		7	7	6	7	7	6
(n =		76	28	48	76	28	48)

*Wives' definitions used.

Table 9.6 Men: Smoking Patterns at Twelve Months

MRC Categories*		All	Occupational Non-manual	Manual	Age —44	45-54	55+
			%	%	%	%	%
Category 1	non-smoker	42	54	35	15	50	43
Category 2	moderate	8	14	4	8	5	14
Category 3		22	21	23	8	24	29
Category 4	heavy	13	4	19	38	10	5
Category 5		14	7	19	31	12	10
(n =		76	28	48	13	42	21)

*Wives' definitions used.

Table 9.7 Wives' Expectations about Husbands' Smoking Habits[*]

Husband at twelve months	Optimistic	Pessimistic
	%	%
Non-smoker	80	18
Moderate smoker	20	41
Heavy smoker	0	41
(n =	20	34)

*Wives' definitions used.

Table 9.8 Wives' Smoking Habits before Husbands' Infarction[*]

Husband at twelve months	Non-smoker	Heavy smoker
	%	%
Non-smoker	49	20
Moderate smoker	25	40
Heavy smoker	25	40
(n =	35	20)

*Wives' definitions used.

Table 10.1: Wife's Health in 12 months

	Husbands' Occupation				Husbands' Age				
	I, II	IIIa	III	IV, V	−44	45-49	50-54	55-59	All
	%	%	%	%	%	%	%	%	%
Consulted GP	48	57	75	56	85	48	48	76	62
Illness, no consultation	14	0	6	13	8	10	10	10	9
No illness	38	43	19	31	6	43	43	14	29
(n =	21	7	32	16	13	21	21	21	76)

	Wife's Age				
	−44	45-49	50-54	55-59	All
	%	%	%	%	%
Consulted GP	64	67	57	62	62
Illness, no consultation	4	13	7	15	9
No illness	31	21	36	23	29
(n =	25	24	14	13	76)

Table 10.2: Wives' views on impact of illness and action taken related to husbands social class and age

Wife Reports Husband's Food	Husbands' Occupation				Husbands Age				
	I, II	IIIa	III	IV, V	−49	45-49	50-54	55-59	All
	%	%	%	%	%	%	%	%	%
Changed	67	57	50	44	46	57	67	43	54
Changed Temporarily	0	14	9	19	15	5	5	14	9
No Change	33	29	41	31	31	38	29	43	36
n.a.	0	0	0	6	8	0	0	0	1

Wife Reports Money to be									
A major problem	14	29	19	50	31	24	19	29	25
Intermediate	5	0	34	19	38	10	33	5	20
Not major problem	81	71	47	31	31	67	48	67	55
(n =	21	7	32	16	13	21	21	21	76)

Table 10.2 (Continued)

Wife Considers her Responsibilities	Husbands' Occupation				Husbands' Age				
	I, II	IIIa	III	IV,V	—44	45-49	50-54	55-59	All
	%	%	%	%	%	%	%	%	%
Increased	57	57	34	56	48	38	52	52	47
Temporarily/ Intermediate	14	14	6	19	8	24	10	5	12
No change	29	29	59	25	46	38	38	43	41
Husband's Household Tasks									
Wife reports taken over	76	57	56	56	38	76	62	62	62
Temporarily taken over	10	0	9	19	15	10	19	0	11
No change	14	43	34	25	46	14	19	38	28
Wife Reports Sexual Intercourse									
More frequent	5	0	0	0	0	0	0	5	1
Same as before	5	29	25	13	46	24	10	0	17
Less frequent	43	0	34	44	38	29	48	29	36
n.a.	48	71	41	44	15	48	43	67	46
Wife Considers Husband's Personality									
Changed lastingly	62	43	63	69	46	62	86	48	62
Changed temporarily	5	0	6	6	8	5	0	9	5
No change	33	57	31	25	46	33	14	43	33
Wife Reports Husband Confides									
Very readily in her	43	57	25	13	23	33	29	33	30
With some reservations	19	0	28	19	31	24	24	10	21
Decidedly does not	38	43	47	63	38	43	48	57	47
n.a.	0	0	0	6	8	0	0	0	1
(n =	21	7	32	16	13	21	21	21	76)

n.a. = not asked or not applicable.

Table 10.2 (Continued)

Wife Reports Husbands' Work Habits	Husband's Occupation				Husbands' Age				
	I, II	IIIa	III	IV, V	−44	45-49	50-54	55-59	All
	%	%	%	%	%	%	%	%	%
Still changed	48	43	50	25	31	62	43	33	43
Temporarily changed	14	14	0	13	15	0	10	10	8
No change	24	29	41	25	31	33	33	29	32
n.a.	14	14	9	38	23	5	14	29	17
Wife Thinks Possible Recurrence									
Worries husband	19	29	28	25	38	24	14	29	25
d.k. or reservations	43	43	44	50	23	57	48	43	45
Husband not worried	33	29	22	13	23	14	29	29	24
n.a.	5	0	6	13	15	5	10	0	7
Wife Thinks Husband Consults GP									
Adequately	57	43	59	44	62	48	48	62	54
Intermediate/ reservations	19	14	6	25	0	14	19	19	14
Not adequately	24	43	34	31	38	38	33	19	32
Wife Discussed Husband's Illness with G.P.									
Adequately	33	43	22	50	31	29	29	43	33
At beginning only	10	14	6	0	8	0	19	0	7
Not at all	57	43	72	50	62	71	52	57	61
(n =	21	7	32	16	13	21	21	21	76)

Table 10.2 (Continued)

Wife Considers Advice to Husband	Husbands' Occupation				Husbands' Age				
	I, II	IIIa	III	IV, V	—44	45-49	50-54	55-59	All
	%	%	%	%	%	%	%	%	%
Practicable	71	57	69	60	50	62	71	76	66
Practicable in part only	29	43	31	27	42	38	29	19	31
Not practicable	0	0	0	13	8	0	0	5	3
Wife Considers Husband Follows									
All medical advice	71	57	38	40	8	52	62	57	49
In part only	24	43	53	40	67	33	38	38	41
Advice not followed	5	0	9	20	25	14	0	6	9
Wife's Role in Medical Régime									
Appears moderate	81	43	59	80	50	81	75	57	68
Appears extreme (positive)	5	43	25	20	25	5	19	33	20
Appears extreme (negative)	14	14	16	0	25	14	5	10	12
Wife Considers Medical Services									
Were adequate	67	43	75	63	62	62	67	76	67
With reservations	33	43	19	25	31	19	33	24	26
Were not adequate	0	14	6	6	8	14	0	0	5
n.a.	0	0	0	6	0	5	0	0	1
(n =	21	7	32	16	13	21	21	21	76)

n.a. = not asked or not applicable

Table 10.3: Wife Considers Help in Employment*

	Husbands' Occupation				Husbands' Age				
	I, II	IIIa	III	IV, V	−44	45-49	50-54	55-59	All
	%	%	%	%	%	%	%	%	%
Was adequate	55	50	50	33	50	45	50	53	49
With reservations	33	0	23	44	20	30	22	33	27
Was not adequate	11	50	26	22	30	25	27	13	24
(n =	18	6	30	9	10	20	18	15	63)

*n = 63 men who returned to work.

Table 11.1: Outcome at 12 months

'A' — husband working and wife considers illness over	29
'B' — husband working but wife considers illness not over	27
'C' — husband not working	20
TOTAL	76

Table 11.2: Outcome at 12 months by husbands' age

	39	40-44	45-49	50-54	55-59
	%	%	%	%	%
A	40	13	47	34	43
B	20	25	43	53	19
C	40	63	10	14	38
(n =	5	8	21	21	21)

The figures in Tables 11.3 to 12.6 are percentages of relevant totals for Non-manual/Manual families with outcomes 'A', 'B' and 'C'. Percentages in some tables add up to more than 100 because more than one category may apply

It is appreciated that numbers in 'B' and 'C' Non-manual are very small. However, if these two outcomes are combined, the contrast with 'A' Non-manual is in the required direction.

Table 11.3: Outcome at 12 months by husband's age and occupation

Age	Non-manual			Manual		
	A	B	C	A	B	C
	%	%	%	%	%	%
−39) 40-44)	13	11	0	7	11	43
45-49) 50-54)	60	77	0	57	72	31
55-59	26	11	100	35	16	25
(n =	15	9	4	14	18	16)

Table 11.4: Husband's Household Tasks

	Non-manual			All	Manual			All
	A	B	C	NM	A	B	C	M
	%	%	%	%	%	%	%	%
Wife reports taken over	60	100	50	71	42	77	43	56
Temporarily taken over	13	0	0	7	14	0	25	12
No change	26	0	50	21	42	22	31	31
(n =	15	9	4	28	14	18	16	48)

Table 11.5: Wife Reports Husband's Work Habits

	Non-manual			Manual		
	A	B	C	A	B	C
	%	%	%	%	%	%
Changed	67	33	n.a.	71	47	n.a.
Changed temporarily	0	44	n.a.	0	5	n.a.
No change	33	22	n.a.	24	47	n.a.
(n =	15	9		14	18	)

Table 11.6: Wife's Paid Employment

	Non-manual			Manual		
	A	B	C	A	B	C
	%	%	%	%	%	%
None	46	77	0	28	22	20
Normally full-time	20	11	75	57	16	53
Normally part-time	33	11	25	14	61	26
(n =	15	9	4	14	18	16)

Table 11.7: Wife's Expectations at Crisis

	Non-manual			Manual		
	A	B	C	A	B	C
	%	%	%	%	%	%
Very favourable	53	44	50	14	28	19
Intermediate	47	44	50	72	44	38
Very unfavourable	0	12	0	14	28	43
(n =	15	0	4	14	18	16)

Table 11.8: Areas of Potential Stress — Total Assessed

	Non-manual			Manual		
	A	B	C	A	B	C
	%	%	%	%	%	%
Number of areas = 0–2	67	33	25	43	28	19
Number of areas = 3–5	33	67	75	57	72	81
(n =	15	9	4	14	18	16)

Table 11.9: Specific Areas of Potential Stress

	Non-manual			Manual		
	A	B	C	A	B	C
	%	%	%	%	%	%
Husband's pre-infarction health	0	22	25	21	11	44
Husband's work	33	67	75	43	67	75
Husband's personality	80	78	100	86	89	81
Nuclear family	53	78	50	43	67	75
Network	33	44	50	50	56	75
(n =	15	9	4	14	18	16)

Table 11.10: Husband's Position in Family of Origin

	Non-manual			Manual			All
	A	B	C	A	B	C	
	%	%	%	%	%	%	%
Eldest	13	22	0	7	17	44	20
Intermediate	33	45	75	71	56	25	47
Youngest	47	33	0	21	28	19	28
Only	7	0	25	0	0	12	5
(n =	15	9	4	14	18	16	76)

Table 11.11: Wife's Position in Family of Origin

	Non-manual			Manual			All
	A	B	C	A	B	C	
	%	%	%	%	%	%	%
Eldest	27	22	0	50	17	12	24
Intermediate	33	33	50	22	50	50	40
Youngest	34	44	0	22	28	25	28
Only	7	0	50	7	6	12	9
(n =	15	9	4	14	18	16	76)

Table 12.1: Number of Sources of Help Reported at Crisis

	Non-manual			Manual			All
	A	B	C	A	B	C	
	%	%	%	%	%	%	%
0 source	7	0	0	0	6	0	3
1 "	20	33	50	36	28	44	33
2 "	27	44	25	36	39	50	38
3+ "	47	22	25	29	28	6	26
(n =	15	9	4	14	18	16	76)

Table 12.2: Number of Sources of Help Reported in Post-Infarction Year

	Non-manual			Manual			All
	A	B	C	A	B	C	
	%	%	%	%	%	%	%
0 source	13	11	25	0	22	13	13
1 "	47	67	50	64	44	69	57
2 "	20	22	25	21	22	19	21
3+ "	20	0	0	14	11	0	9
(n =	15	9	4	14	18	16	76)

Table 12.3: Helpers Reported At Crisis

	Non-manual			Manual			All
	A	B	C	A	B	C	
	%	%	%	%	%	%	%
Children	67	56	25	71	67	44	59
Wife's kin	53	44	0	64	39	50	47
Husband's kin	33	22	50	29	44	19	32
'Others'	73	78	100	43	50	50	49
(n =	15	9	4	14	18	16	76)

Table 12.4: Helpers Reported in Post-Infarction Year

	Non-manual			Manual			All
	A	B	C	A	B	C	
	%	%	%	%	%	%	%
Children	40	44	25	79	61	50	54
Wife's kin	40	22	0	36	28	19	28
Husband's kin	20	11	25	21	22	19	20
'Others'	40	33	25	7	11	13	20
(n =	15	9	4	14	18	16	76)

Table 12.5 Anticipated Lay Consultants

	Outcome	Non-manual			Manual			All
		A	B	C	A	B	C	
		%	%	%	%	%	%	%
Children		13	11	25	14	22	13	16
Husband		47	67	50	21	28	13	33
Wife's kin		40	33	0	43	39	63	42
Husband's kin		7	11	0	14	11	16	9
'Others' —								
professional		20	11	50	7	6	13	13
non-professional		13	22	0	14	11	25	16
No consultant		7	0	0	7	6	6	5
(n =		15	9	4	14	18	16	76)

Table 12.6 Lay Consultants reported at 12 months

	Outcome	Non-manual			Manual			All
		A	B	C	A	B	C	
		%	%	%	%	%	%	%
Children		20	11	0	43	28	6	21
Husband		87	44	50	21	39	25	43
Wife's kin		13	22	0	29	33	38	26
Husband's kin		0	11	25	21	17	0	11
'Others' — all								
non-professional		27	22	50	14	6	6	16
No consultant		7	22	25	14	28	44	24
(n =		15	9	4	14	18	16	76)

Table 13.1 Outcome at four years (100% = 88)

	Age					
	−39	40-44	45-49	50-54	55-59	Total
Alive and interviewed	5%	10%	18%	20%	14%	67%
Alive not interviewed (not in area)			2%	2%	2%	6%
Dead from heart disease		5%	2%	2%	13%	22%
Dead from other cause					2%	2%
Not traced	1%			1%		2%
TOTAL	6%	15%	22%	25%	31%	99%

Table 13.2 Symptoms at four years (100% = 59)

	Angina	Other Heart Symptoms
Yes — Severe	10%	10%
Yes — Not Severe	56%	27%
No	34%	63%

Table 13.3 Number of men with further episodes of illness during four years (requiring medical care) (100% = 59)

	None	Requiring Hospital Admission	Treated at Home
Associated with heart	73%	17%	10% (100%)
Other illness (excluding minor)	61%	17%	22% (100%)

Table 13.4 Treatment at four years

On treatment for heart condition	51%
On treatment for other conditions	14%

Table 13.5 Time off work due to illness (100% = 53)

	None	Less than 3 months	4-6 months	Greater than 6 months
Heart conditions	75%	11%	11%	3% (100%)
Other conditions	66%	25%	8	1% (100%)

Table 13.6 Employment position at four years (100% = 59)

Employed	90%
Unemployed	2%
Retired	—
Not Working Due to Illness	8%
	(100%)

Table 13.7 Nature of employment (100% = 54)

Same work as prior to infarction	57%
Same work as returned to after infarction	17%
More than one change of work	26%
	(100%)

Table 13.8 Hours of work at four years compared to before infarction (100% = 53)

Same	57%
Less	43%
More	—
	(100%)

Table 13.9 Participation in activities at four years (100% = 59)

	Physical Activities	Social Activities
Less	46%	49%
Same	32%	44%
More	22%	7%
	(100%)	(100%)

Table 13.10 Smoking patterns after infarction; position at four years (100% = 59)

Non-smoker	Pipe smoker	$<$14/day	15-24/day	25-49/day	50 or more/day
42%	14%	10%	14%	17%	3%

Table 13.11 Attitude towards illness (100% = 58)

Illness finished	31%
Illness still a present problem	31%
Illness over but thought at back of mind	38%

Table 13.12 Achievement of stable pattern of life (100% = 58)

By 4 months	15%
By 9 months	52%
By 14 months	71%
By 2 years	84%
By 4 years	88%
Never	12%

Table 13.13 Attitudes to illness and present health (100% = 58)

Entirely positive	25%
Mixed	21%
Entirely negative	54%

INDEX